The Nurse Mentor's
Hand

The Nurse Mentor's Handbook

Supporting Students in Clinical Practice

SECOND EDITION

Danny Walsh

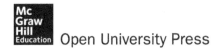

Mc Graw Hill Education Open University Press

Open University Press
McGraw-Hill Education
McGraw-Hill House
Shoppenhangers Road
Maidenhead
Berkshire
England
SL6 2QL

email: enquiries@openup.co.uk
world wide web: www.openup.co.uk

and Two Penn Plaza, New York, NY 10121-2289, USA

First published 2010
First published in this second edition 2014

A catalogue record of this book is available from the British Library

ISBN-13: 978-0-335-26318-9
ISBN-10: 0-335-26318-6
eISBN: 978-0-335-26319-6

Library of Congress Cataloging-in-Publication Data
CIP data applied for

Typeset by Aptara Inc., India

Praise for this book

"This book is essential reading for newly qualified nurses intending to develop their professional skills by becoming mentors. Well written in accessible language the book progresses logically and comprehensively providing a comprehensive resource for both novice and experienced mentors."

Dr David Howard, Associate Professor, School of Health and Social Care,
The University of Lincoln, UK

Praise for the first edition

"The book is user-friendly and easy to read. It is informative and very relevant in the current climate where there is a need to ensure that education and practice work together in the interest of mentors, students, and practitioners."

Lynne Walsh, School of Health Science, Swansea University, UK

"This book is an excellent resource for becoming mentors, new mentors, and existing mentors. It is a comprehensive guide to mentoring under NMC regulations, and there is much here that is relevant to all those that mentor in practice settings.

The available evidence informs and guides the text, but this is a handbook for action: there is a wealth of practical advice and activities that will enhance mentor practice and enrich the clinical area as a learning environment."

Brian James, Senior Teaching Fellow, University of Stirling, UK

"The importance of the role of the mentor in the education and development of healthcare professionals who are fit to practice is well recognised. This book, which focuses on the role as it applies to nursing, is a timely and complementary addition to the growing 'pool' of available literature on this subject.

The book offers mentors and 'would-be mentors' a cogent approach built on practical experience and a rational synthesis constructed from the field of relevant literature. The author uses 'real-world' anecdotal student comments to illustrate the points made, thus providing valuable insight into the student perspective. Throughout the book the author does not shy away from contentious areas and while it is fair to say that there is usually more than one possible approach available, these issues are addressed in an open and forthright manner that provides the reader with a thought-through response.

The author's style is easy to read, uses accessible language, and offers the reader plenty of practical advice about this demanding role. The author has also addressed contemporary developments and has linked the text firmly to Professional Body requirements. The above features contribute to making a book that is both readable and informative."

Sylvia Hepworth, University of Huddersfield, UK

Contents

Figures

Acknowledgements

I am hugely indebted to Sylvia Hepworth whose wisdom and experience I have called upon many times in the production of this book; as far as mentors go, there could be no better.

I am also grateful to Clare Sobieraj for her helpful contributions and support during the process of writing this book. The advice and contributions of my colleague Fran Maplethorpe have also been invaluable. Special thanks also go to Diane Ramm who has drawn on her considerable experience to write an important section detailing the key principles of teaching clinical skills, and to Chris Craggs who updated the section relating to students with disability.

Many of the mentor and student quotes used within were drawn from various student evaluations from a range of nursing courses nationally. Many were also sent to me anonymously, so to persons unknown I am especially grateful. Some narratives were recollected on request specifically for this book and I am grateful to these contributors: S. Bettles, A. Hurrell, N. Raybould, Y. Potter, C. Burrows, Z. Mabandla, G. Helme, and I. Trueman.

Finally, my gratitude goes to Rachel Crookes, the senior commissioning editor for Nursing and Health at McGraw-Hill, whose encouragement and guidance have both kept me going and enhanced this book.

Introduction

Arguably the most important aspect of nursing and midwifery training is the clinical placement during which nurses learn and practise their many skills in the real world. The most important factor underpinning a good placement is the mentor who works with the student. All nurses have a duty, through their professional code of conduct, to pass on their knowledge and to mentor students – and this book is a guide to doing just that. This second edition of *The Nurse Mentor's Handbook* embraces recent changes in nurse education such as the revised Nursing and Midwifery Council pre–registration competencies (NMC 2010). There has also been an increased emphasis upon evidence-based practice and electronic portfolios. This new edition also re-emphasises the importance of support mechanisms for the mentor in practice, at a time when nurse education providers are trying a varied range of systems to achieve this.

Who is this book for?

The purpose of the book is to examine the role of the nurse acting as mentor to pre-registration student nurses in the light of the mentor standards and outcomes as set out by the Nursing and Midwifery Council (NMC 2008a). The book is intended primarily for those qualified nurses undertaking mentorship courses but will also be of value to qualified mentors as a guide to good practice. It will also be useful to those undertaking mentorship in other related health and social care settings such as occupational therapy, physiotherapy, social work, and operating departments. Their professional standards might vary but as with midwives, the mentoring elements will be transferable.

What this book covers

Since 2007, to become a mentor a nurse must have been qualified for at least one year and then undertake a mentorship course during which they must demonstrate evidence of achievement of the NMC mentor standards and outcomes. The outcomes themselves and the relevant policy context are discussed in Chapter 1. The achievement of the outcomes by budding mentors will be examined in Chapter 7, where a range of ideas for meeting each competence are discussed and the evidence that can be used to demonstrate such achievement is outlined. The beginning of each chapter includes a box highlighting those domains and outcomes that are relevant to that chapter.

Chapter 2 'The effective mentor' examines the role of the mentor generally, trying to capture the essence of what it takes to be a good mentor. It examines some key principles of mentorship, including effective working relationships, communication, and the ability to create and manage learning opportunities. The chapter also looks at the concept of 'toxic' mentoring and how to audit your mentoring skills.

Chapter 3 'The clinical learning environment' examines the qualities of a good learning environment and also what detracts from it. In any learning environment, many factors affect the learning that takes place, for good and for bad. Readers are asked to reflect upon their own experiences here in order to explore key issues. The chapter also covers the key aspects of competency mapping and how this can be achieved, and explores the range of potential learning opportunities in the clinical environment. Furthermore, the chapter introduces a range of strategies that can help improve the learning environment.

Chapter 4 'Teaching and learning theory' concentrates upon the educational theories that abound, examining them for their usefulness and practical application. Behaviourist, cognitive, and humanist approaches to learning and teaching are explored alongside the concepts of andragogy and pedagogy. The chapter also examines the concept of learning styles and the work of Kolb and Honey and Mumford among others.

Chapter 5 'Teaching in practice' looks at the teaching cycle, planning for teaching, and aims and objectives. Bloom's taxonomy is explored, as is the evaluation of teaching. The chapter also outlines the practicalities and skills of delivering teaching and examines the various teaching methods and resources that are available, giving the mentor a range of strategies to choose from. The value and practice of using learning contracts is also outlined.

Chapter 6 'Assessment: theory and practice reality' focuses upon assessment, examining the process and the theory behind it. From definitions and aims of assessment, it goes on to discuss the cardinal criteria for assessment such as validity and reliability. From a practical point of view, a range of assessment methods are examined which can be used to assess clinical competence, again giving the mentor a range of strategies to choose from.

Chapter 7 'Building a portfolio of evidence' offers guidance on how to build a portfolio and what to put in it. The chapter looks at the portfolios student nurses have to keep and the types of evidence that can be used. It also highlights the importance of reflection. As part of their mentor course, many nurses will also have to compile portfolios of evidence, or in other ways demonstrate evidence of achievement of the mentor outcomes, and the chapter looks at the ways in which this can be done.

Chapter 8 'Helping students survive a placement' provides a summary of good practice in relation to supporting students generally. It also looks at the ways in which mentors can help students with disabilities such as dyslexia and dyscalculia, and support students under stress.

Chapter 9 'Supporting failing students' examines the work of Kathleen Duffy and colleagues, who identified that mentors were 'failing to fail' students for various reasons. This study, its evidence and implications are examined in detail before outlining a strategy for fair and objective support for a failing student. The implications for professional (and other) accountability are made clear. Particular emphasis is placed upon the difficult area of assessing a student's 'attitude'. The value and practice of reflection in nurse training is explored. The chapter outlines good practice guidelines for mentors and suggests ways in which the mentor can help the student get the best out of their placement.

Chapter 10 focuses on 'Maintaining ongoing competence and developing as a mentor'. The NMC (2006) *Standards to Support Learning and Assessment in Practice* dictate that mentors must demonstrate their ongoing competence. This will be assessed via a triennial review at which the mentor will have to provide evidence that they have met the NMC criteria and requirements. This chapter examines those 'requirements' and provides a range of strategies relating to how they can be met. The chapter also looks at the evidence mentors could generate in relation to these strategies to demonstrate updating and build a portfolio of ongoing competence. The role of sign-off mentors and the future of nurse mentorship is also examined.

Quotes and narratives

The chapter themes are illustrated in part by quotes and narratives from students in training and mentors. These are real comments and describe the student's raw concerns. It is the kind of feedback straight from the horse's mouth that we should all be gathering and acting upon. The importance of the role of mentors in pre-registration nurse education cannot be underestimated, a point reiterated and evidenced throughout this book and one that these quotes highlight in particular.

Professional support

The most widely used definition of mentor in this context is that given by the NMC (2006), which states that a mentor is essentially a registered nurse who, having met the requirements for the mentor standard, 'facilitates learning and supervises and assesses students in a practice setting'. As definitions go, it is quite succinct but it doesn't do justice to the diversity of roles involved or the range of knowledge and skills required to meet it. That nurses do not get any 'time out' for mentoring a student is hard to reconcile with the requirements of the role. Compared with other professions, we are the poor relation here. In their *Standards and Guidance for Mentors* document (AODP 2006), the Association of Operating Department Practitioners recommends that mentors have four hours a week protected time per student. This is to allow them 'sufficient time to provide regular supervision, including assessment and feedback'. Social workers receive enhanced payments for mentoring students. Occupational therapists are in the same boat as nurses. Their *Code of Ethics and Professional Conduct* (College of Occupational Therapists 2005) asks that they make a commitment to the education of students in the workplace, having a 'professional responsibility to provide educational opportunities for occupational therapy students' (5.5). For this role, like nurses, there is no protected time or any extra remuneration, they simply have to try and put aside time for a weekly supervision session with their student. The NMC *Standards to Support Learning and Assessment in Practice* (2006) state that mentors 'will need time, when undertaking work with a student, to be able to explain, question, assess performance and provide feedback to the student in a meaningful way' (NMC 2006, p. 30). The document goes on to state as an NMC requirement that sign-off mentors should be allowed one hour a week per student. Given the professional responsibility involved here, this is derisory. The document has little to offer non-sign-off mentors who must balance their clinical and managerial duties with mentoring students.

In 2009, the NMC began a review of pre-registration nurse education with the aim of developing a teaching, learning, and assessment framework suitable for the future of an all-degree profession (NMC 2009). As part of this process, a practice educator facilitator workshop identified 10 priority areas of concern, one of which was mentorship. It raised the question, should all nurses be mentors? An acknowledgement perhaps that a significant number of nurses have far too little time to be effective mentors, but it also acknowledged a lack of funding for mentorship and, most tellingly, lamented the lack of value attributed to the status of mentors. The nursing professional body should recognise the importance of mentoring by introducing protected time, if not financial reward for undertaking the role. The theory side of training has been elevated to degree status, but the practice side of training is arguably more deserving of elevation and status, and this can be achieved in part by recognising and giving real value to the role of the mentor.

Benefits of mentoring

As nurses we have a professional duty to become mentors as set out in the Code of Conduct: 'You must facilitate students and others to develop their competence' (NMC 2008b). But it is a role nurses should wish to embrace, as it is by no means just one-way traffic. Here are just a few of the tangible reasons for becoming a mentor:

- Increased job satisfaction
- Increased professional role
- Involvement with the higher education provider
- Being updated by and learning from the students

- Developing teaching skills
- Adding to personal profile/CV
- Mentoring skills useful in other areas such as management
- Gratitude of the students, increased self-esteem
- Opportunity to impact upon curriculum and nurse training
- Maintaining the standards of your own profession
- Helping to protect the public

Students' views

Here are a selection of student reflections suggesting that good mentors are highly valued.

Second-year student on medical ward

What stood out for me was working closely with motivated mentors who were willing to share the wealth of their knowledge despite the pressures of their hectic shifts.

Third-year student on surgical ward

Every member of the team was approachable and helpful. I was made to feel valued at all times. Nothing was too much trouble for my mentor and associate mentor.

Third-year student on emergency assessment unit

Very welcoming staff made the placement very enjoyable. I have gained valuable knowledge and skills from excellent mentors. They put lots of effort into the teaching despite the busy workload.

First-year student on medical acute placement

My mentor gave me plenty of opportunity to take part in clinical skills and I didn't feel pressured to contribute if I felt I couldn't do it. Everyone tried to make me feel welcome and get the best experience I could.

Third-year student on forensic mental health placement

I think what makes a good mentor is one that takes an interest in their students' learning and gets them involved. Somebody you can look up to in

(continued)

terms of practice and say to yourself I want to be like that. Somebody who can tell you what you don't do well in such a way as to make it not feel like a criticism but an opportunity. I've been very lucky.

First-year mental health student

This placement was a remarkable experience and the credit is due to my mentor.

Summary

- This introduction has hinted at both the diversity and importance of the role of the mentor and this will become even more apparent in the following chapters.

- It is well documented that mentors are pivotal in ensuring a student nurse has a good placement experience, and this view is supported by the students quoted in this book.

- The NMC standards for mentors define the mentor role and describe what the mentor has to do and be in order to be effective.

These standards, their history, and their policy context are explored next in Chapter 1.

Further reading

Andrews, M. and Wallis, M. (1999) Mentorship in nursing: a literature review, *Journal of Advanced Nursing*, 29(1): 201–7. Despite being published in 1999, this is a useful article because it helps to set the scene for many of the themes to be discussed later. It allows us to reflect upon concerns raised then and those apparent now and ponder how far we have progressed (or not).

Atkins, S. and Williams, A. (1995) Registered nurses' experience of mentoring undergraduate nursing students, *Journal of Advanced Nursing*, 21(5): 1006–15.

Field, D.E. (2004) Moving from novice to expert – the value of learning in clinical practice: a literature review, *Nurse Education Today*, 24(7): 560–5.

Pulsford, D., Boit, K. and Owen, S. (2002) Are mentors ready to make a difference? A survey of mentors' attitudes towards nurse education, *Nurse Education Today*, 22(6): 439–46.

Watson, S. (2004) Mentor preparation: reasons for undertaking the course and expectations of the candidates, *Nurse Education Today*, 24(1): 30–40.

References

Association of Operating Department Practitioners (AODP) (2006) *Qualifications Framework for Mentors Supporting Learners in Practice: Standards and guidance for mentors and practice placements in support of pre-registration diploma of higher education in operating department practice provision.* Wilmslow: AODP.

College of Occupational Therapists (2005) *Code of Ethics and Professional Conduct.* London: College of Occupational Therapists.

Nursing and Midwifery Council (NMC) (2006) *Standards to Support Learning and Assessment in Practice: NMC standards for mentors, practice teachers and teachers.* London: NMC.

Nursing and Midwifery Council (NMC) (2008a) *Standards to Support Learning and Assessment in Practice: NMC standards for mentors, practice teachers and teachers,* 2nd edn. London: NMC.

Nursing and Midwifery Council (NMC) (2008b) *The Code: Standards of conduct, performance and ethics for nurses and midwives.* London: NMC.

Nursing and Midwifery Council (NMC) (2009) *NMC Review of Pre-registration Nurse Education,* Bulletin 3. London: NMC. Available at: www.nmc.org.uk/aArticle-aspx?ArticleID=3566 [accessed 5 January 2010].

Nursing and Midwifery Council (NMC) (2010) *Standards for Pre-registration Nursing Education.* London: NMC. Available at: http://standards.nmc-uk.org/Published Documents/Standards%20for%20pre-registration%20nursing%20education%2016082010.pdf [accessed 2 March 2014].

1 The Nursing and Midwifery Council standards and outcomes for mentors and their policy context

Key points

- The NMC mentor standards act as a template for good mentorship, highlighting the important role of mentors in nurse education

- The mentor standards are born of a desire to re-emphasise the practice element of nurse education

- The mentor standards can be mapped to the NHS Knowledge and Skills Framework

- The NMC sets out clear principles and requirements for placements

The aim of this book is to examine in depth the NMC domains or standards for mentors. However, before examining their practical application and the 'how to' aspects of mentoring, it is useful to look back briefly at how the standards have come into being and understand the context in which they have developed. The chapter also looks at mentorship and the NHS Knowledge and Skills Framework, and the sometimes apparently chaotic nature of mentorship!

History and context of mentorship standards

In 1999, the Department of Health (DH) published a strategy for nursing entitled *Making a Difference*. The document was critical of the abilities of newly trained nurses on the previous Project 2000 curriculum: 'Evidence suggests that in recent years students completing training have not been equipped at the point of qualification with the full range of clinical skills they need' (DH 1999: para. 2.26, p. 14). The strategy also heavily stressed the importance of practice placements in nurse education, as highlighted in the quotes on the next page.

'Provision of clinical placements is a vital part of the education process'

'We want to get practical skills into education programmes from the start'

'We want higher quality and longer placements in a genuinely supportive learning environment'

'We are determined to enhance the status of those who provide practice based training' (DH 1999: para. 4.11, p. 27)

The Department of Health wanted to ensure that nurses were 'fit for purpose', having the necessary skills, knowledge, and ability to provide the best care.

During the same year, the UK Central Council for Nursing, Midwifery and Health Visiting (UKCC) published its review of nurse education entitled *Fitness for Practice* (UKCC 1999). Essentially, this document stressed the need to emphasise the role of the mentor/teacher in the practice setting and reiterated the belief that practice experience was crucial to nurse education. The report also acknowledged the need for higher education institutions (HEIs) and health service providers to formalise the preparation of mentors for nurses in training. The current standards for mentors and nurse teachers ultimately derive from this review. The other significant change was the accreditation of 50% given to the achievement of clinical practice outcomes, thus raising the status of the clinical aspect of training and underlining the need for credible mentor preparation programmes.

Subsequent reports such as *Placements in Focus* (ENB/DH 2001) confirmed this message. Partnership between the National Health Service (NHS) and HEIs was stressed and both became responsible for providing and supporting clinical placements. The partnership between the clinical areas and the HEIs is crucial because, as Hand (2006) points out, skill without knowledge fosters unsafe practice and knowledge without skill fosters incompetence.

How robust do you consider the partnership between your own clinical area and the university and how could this be improved upon?

The NMC framework to support learning and assessment in practice

The NMC mentor standards or domains describe the outcomes nurses must attain to become mentors to student nurses. These outcomes were published by the NMC in the document *Standards to Support Learning and Assessment in Practice* (NMC 2006). This document also sets the standards and outcomes for practice teachers, and teachers of midwives, nurses, and specialist community public health nurses. The document introduces a framework for the development of nurse teachers and identifies four key stages:

Stage 1   NMC registrant

Stage 2   Mentor

Stage 3   Practice teacher

Stage 4   Teacher

Underpinning this framework are five principles for supporting students who are working towards NMC recordable qualifications. These dictate that the mentor/assessor must:

A.   Be on the same part of the register as that which the student is working towards

B.   Have developed their knowledge and skills beyond registration

C.   Hold professional qualifications equal to or at a higher level than that which the students are working towards

D.   Have been prepared for their role and met the NMC outcomes for such

E.   Record any NMC-approved teaching qualifications on the register

This developmental framework also identifies eight domains for each stage:

• Establishing effective working relationships

• Facilitation of learning

• Assessment and accountability

• Evaluation of learning

• Creating an environment for learning

• Context of practice

• Evidence-based practice

• Leadership

These domains were a revision of those previously published by the NMC in 2004 as *Standards for the Preparation of Teachers of Nurses, Midwives and Specialist Community Public Health Nurses*. The 2004 standard of 'Role modelling' was replaced with the domain of 'Leadership'. They were also modified slightly in 2008 in the second edition of *Standards to Support Learning and Assessment in Practice* (NMC 2008).

Mentor domains

The mentor domains (or standards as they were called) represent the competencies and outcomes for mentors. Each domain is broken down into several outcomes:

Establish effective working relationships

- Demonstrate an understanding of factors that influence how students integrate into practice

- Provide ongoing and constructive support to facilitate transition from one learning environment to another

- Have effective professional and interprofessional working relationships to support learning for entry to the register

Facilitation of learning

- Use knowledge of the student's stage of learning to select appropriate learning opportunities to meet their individual needs

- Facilitate selection of appropriate learning strategies to integrate learning from practice and academic experiences

- Support students in critically reflecting upon their learning experiences in order to enhance future learning

Assessment and accountability

- Foster professional growth, personal development, and accountability through support of students in practice

- Demonstrate a breadth of understanding of assessment strategies and the ability to contribute to the total assessment process as part of the teaching team

- Provide constructive feedback to students and assist them in identifying future learning needs and actions. Manage failing students so they may either enhance their performance and capabilities for safe and effective practice, or be able to understand their failure and the implications of this for their future

- Be accountable for confirming that students have met, or not met, the NMC competencies in practice. As a sign-off mentor, confirm that students have met, or not met, the NMC standards of competence in practice and are capable of safe and effective practice

(continued)

Evaluation of learning

- Contribute to evaluation of student learning and assessment experiences – proposing aspects for change as a result of such evaluation
- Participate in self and peer evaluation to facilitate personal development, and contribute to the development of others

Creating an environment for learning

- Support students to identify both learning needs and experiences that are appropriate to their level of learning
- Use a range of learning experiences, involving patients, clients, carers, and the professional team, to meet the defined learning needs
- Identify aspects of the learning environment that could be enhanced, negotiating with others to make appropriate changes
- Act as a resource to facilitate personal and professional developments of others

Context of practice

- Contribute to the development of an environment in which effective practice is fostered, implemented, evaluated, and disseminated
- Set and maintain professional boundaries that are sufficiently flexible for providing interprofessional care
- Initiate and respond to practice developments to ensure safe and effective care is achieved and an effective learning environment is maintained

Evidence-based practice

- Identify and apply research- and evidence-based practice to their area of practice
- Contribute to strategies to increase or review the evidence base used to support practice
- Support students in applying an evidence base to their own practice

Leadership

- Plan a series of learning experiences that will meet students' defined learning needs
- Be an advocate for students to support them accessing learning opportunities that meet their individual needs – involving a range of other professionals, patients, clients, and carers

(continued)

- Prioritise work to accommodate support of students within their practice

- Provide feedback about the effectiveness of learning and assessment in practice

Ideas for the achievement of these outcomes are explored in Chapter 7, 'Building a portfolio of evidence', as most mentorship courses require would-be mentors to provide evidence that they meet these standards.

Knowledge and Skills Framework

The mentor standards and each of the sub-clauses can be used at appraisal, as they closely reflect many of the NHS Knowledge and Skills Framework (KSF) dimensions (DH 2004) upon which many job role descriptors are based. Each dimension has four levels to help identify and aid progression. They define the knowledge and skills nurses and other NHS staff need to perform their roles. The duty of all nurses to facilitate students is also enshrined in this framework, and the role of mentoring is thus often linked to promotion and career progression. Indeed, the purpose of the KSF is to guide staff development and provide a framework for appraisal and review and hence career progression. Many of the mentor domains and sub-clauses relate directly to the KSF dimensions and to demonstrate achievement and competence in key KSF areas, it is a good exercise to map the mentor standards to these. The key dimensions are Communication, People and Personal Development, Health, Safety and Security, Service Improvement, Quality, and Equality and Diversity. The NHS Staff Council (2013) recently reviewed the KSF in order to simplify it, and this review added the dimension of Leadership and Management. The original KSF also had dimensions specific to Health and Wellbeing, Estates and Facilities, and several general dimensions including Learning and Development, and these can still be used to guide development. Use a table like that below to map your mentoring knowledge and skills:

KSF dimension	Mentor standard/clause/skills
Communication	
People and Personal Development	
Health, Safety, and Security	
Service Improvement	
Quality	
Equality and Diversity	
Leadership and Management	
Health and Wellbeing	
Estates and Facilities	
Learning and Development	

NMC mentor/placement principles and requirements

There are many broad principles and essential requirements underpinning nurse education and mentorship, the most significant of which are as follows:

- The NMC decrees that nurses must have been qualified for more than one year and demonstrate continuing professional development before they are eligible to become mentors.

- The mentor must hold a professional qualification equal to or higher than that of the students they are mentoring.

- They must have undertaken and passed an NMC-recognised mentor course.

- They must be able to identify and support learning opportunities in their practice area and in interprofessional arenas.

- They must be able to make judgements about a student's level of competence.

While giving direct care to clients, at least 40% of a student's time must be spent being directly or indirectly supervised by a mentor. The NMC suggests that this 'directness' will vary according to the nature of the task, the student's level of competence (as assessed by their mentor), and the need to assess for outcomes or competencies. Thus the level of supervision will reflect the mentor's assessment of the student's degree of competence. The importance of this is highlighted in Chapter 9, 'Supporting failing students', where the accountability of the mentor to the NMC and for ensuring public protection is discussed.

The mentor should have access to a support network and supervision. This is especially so in cases where difficult decisions such as failures are to be made. Other more experienced mentors and sign-off mentors can provide this. There should also be strong links with the university and a named link tutor or practice representative to provide ongoing support.

The NMC recognises that modern nurses are working within an increasingly interprofessional environment and that at times it is pertinent for the student to gain experience of that interprofessional context. An example might be a mental health nurse gaining experience in a learning disability unit to explore dual diagnosis, or an adult nurse spending some time with a mental health team to gain an understanding of depression. Similarly, nurses now routinely interact with a wide range of other professionals in the course of their work, and it is important that they gain an insight into the work and role of these other colleagues.

The concept of sign-off mentors was introduced by the NMC in 2006. These final placement mentors have the responsibility for scrutinising and 'signing off' the student's three years' worth of placement records. This is discussed in more detail in Chapter 10, 'Maintaining competence as a mentor'.

Ongoing achievement record

The document *Standards to Support Learning and Assessment in Practice* (NMC 2006) introduced what was often referred to as the student 'passport'. This is a record of each placement in a book/file that is taken from placement to placement. Since 2007, it has become known as the 'Ongoing Achievement Record' (OAR). This includes the outcomes and comments from previous mentors and placements, and allows opinions to be formed regarding the student's overall progress and to identify any areas of need at the start of each subsequent placement. This enables sign-off mentors to access the student's complete placement record and appraise it and confirm that areas of concern have been addressed. The NMC (2007) state that the OAR is to be used within 5 days of beginning a placement to develop an action plan for that placement, taking account of any prior concerns raised.

Mentor preparation programmes

The NMC requirements for the course to which this book is addressed suggest that it should:

- be at a minimum of Level 2, otherwise known as diploma level, HE intermediate level or SCGF Level 8;
- be a minimum of 10 days in length, of which 5 days are protected learning time;
- include learning in both practice and academic settings;
- have a work-based learning component as a key feature. This often entails acting as an associate mentor or undertaking tasks related to student learning in the workplace as directed by the course locally. Many such tasks are described in later chapters.

The NMC suggests that the course should be completed within 3 months and that up to 100% of the programme can be accredited to prior learning if the student mentor has undertaken similar relevant previous training.

In reality, there are many variations on this course nationally, it being interpreted locally and creatively in many different ways. However, another reality in some areas suggests that many nurses are struggling to secure their 10 days and managing just 5, making up the rest in their own time. For managers, releasing staff is difficult at the best of times and the course should be seen in the light of its predecessor, which in many areas was interpreted as a 3-day course. The NMC had not previously defined a specific mentor course and previous mentor preparation programmes were approved as part of pre-registration and specialist practice qualification programmes, with much national variation.

NMC review of nurse education 2010

The revised *Standards for Pre-registration Nursing Education* (NMC 2010) were born out of a consultation exercise commissioned by the NMC entitled *Nursing; Towards 2015* (Longley et al. 2007). The new standards ushered in an all-degree profession arguing that this was necessary for the future and to 'enable new nurses to work more closely and effectively with other professionals' (NMC 2010, p. 8). The document revised the generic and field-specific competencies for nursing students and also broadened the range of the Essential Skills Clusters, heralding large changes in the associated student placement assessment paperwork. One other departure from tradition was to allow 300 of the 2300 practice hours to be achieved via simulation. The review also consolidated the progression points at the end of years 1 and 2 and attempted to clarify the nature of the concept of 'due regard', stating that other registered healthcare professionals who have been suitably prepared can supervise and contribute towards the assessment of nursing students. The NMC argue that they want to encourage 'flexibility' in who can support and assess nursing students. It states that non-nurse professionals:

• should be suitably prepared;

• may need to undertake part of a NMC mentorship programme;

• must be on the mentor database;

• must undertake annual updating and triennial reviews.

The glossary of terms clarifies the definition of Registered Health Care Professional as 'a member of a profession in the health field that is regulated by a statutory regulator in the UK, such as the NMC, the Health Professions Council and the General Medical Council' (NMC 2010, p. 150).

In another departure from tradition, Section 3 of the review, under Standard 8, 'Assessment', tells us that at progression points 1 and 2 assessment can be by a nurse in any field. At progression point 3, entry to the register, the assessor must be a 'sign-off mentor' nurse on the same part of the register the student is wishing to enter. Additional guidance relating to mentors reminded mentors that student placement assessment records or 'Ongoing Assessment Records' are to be shared between mentors so that student progress can be judged. It also states that mentors should not keep separate student records but enter all comments into the OAR.

Education in chaos!

Many nursing workplaces are stressful and nurses are faced with constant challenges, including lack of time, organisational reform, new technology, an increasingly aware and challenging patient group, high public expectations, bed shortages, cost-saving measures, and increasing non-nursing

(continued)

and administration duties. To this list we must add the almost constant staff shortages that are the source of most care failings for which nurses are often erroneously blamed by politicians. On such a ward, the picture to an outsider might be one of unremitting chaos. Yet in the face of this chaos high standards of care remain and the fact that the above factors do not often undermine the quality of nursing care, is testimony to the professionalism of today's nurses. It can be argued that they are the glue that holds the NHS together.

This scenario also masks the unofficial training that accompanies such a shift, whereby students witness thinking in action, intuitional decision-making, and creative individualised care in the face of daunting constraints. Many examples of learning opportunities could be described if one just sat and watched a shift, noting all that the nurse did on a clipboard. Alongside skilled physical and psychological care tasks are managerial and decision-making skills, assertive and confident practice. Such nurses can see beyond the chaos and achieve Benner's (2001) intuition. Merely being with these nurses is an important learning experience for students. Much key learning takes place almost by osmosis with the student soaking up styles of nursing, ways of reacting and dealing with complex situations amid uncertainty and pressure. Such experience is as beneficial as structured learning and the use of reflection can help to make sense of it.

When students describe how they leant to become a nurse, they usually cite key role models who they have witnessed regularly in such situations. It is the skill of the mentor in allowing the student to participate according to their ability and level in such dynamic and chaotic scenarios that gives the students the opportunity to build personal and professional competence.

The 2012 NHS London examination of nurse mentorship (Robinson et al. 2012) cites Pulsford and co-workers (2002), reminding us that mentors in this study wanted more support from trust managers and more time for mentoring activity, specifically help with managing multiple demands upon their time. This is still the case and serves as a timely reminder that if nursing shortages increase and mentorship is not given time, we may well lose the most important, albeit chaotic, learning experience that students get.

Summary

This chapter has:

- Examined how the mentor standards were born of a desire to enhance the importance of practice placements in nurse education

(continued)

- Stressed the importance of having robust links between placement areas and the higher education institutions providing the nurse education

- Highlighted the eight mentor domains, their outcomes, and links to the NHS Knowledge and Skills Framework

- Examined the NMC requirements and principles for mentors

- Noted that much valuable teaching and mentorship can appear, and often occurs in, an apparently chaotic environment

It is now pertinent to move on to examine in depth the requirements of the first mentor domain of 'Establishing effective working relationships'.

Further reading

www.practicebasedlearning.org

This website 'aims to enhance the quality of student experiences whilst on practice, i.e. work-based placements'. It covers much ground and has a very useful resource section. It has sections which will be useful to all aspects of mentorship and which relate to many chapters in this book.

References

Benner, P. (2001) *From Novice to Expert: Excellence and power in clinical nursing practice*, commemorative edition. Upper Saddle River, NJ: Prentice-Hall Health.

Department of Health (DH) (1999) *Making a Difference*. London: Department of Health.

Department of Health (DH) (2004) *The NHS Knowledge and Skills Framework (NHS KSF) and the Development Review Process*. London: DH.

ENB/Department of Health (ENB/DH) (2001) *Placements in Focus: Guidance for education in practice for health care professions*. London: English National Board for Nursing, Midwifery and Health Visiting/Department of Health.

Hand, H. (2006) Promoting effective teaching and learning in the practice setting, *Nursing Standard*, 20(39): 55–63.

Longley, M., Shaw, C. and Dolan, G. (2007) *Nursing: Towards 2015*. Pontypridd: Welsh Institute of Health and Social Care.

NHS Staff Council (2013) *Simplified KSF*. Available at: www.nhsemployers.org/pay andcontracts/agendaforchange/ksf/simplified-ksf/pages/simplifiedksf.aspx [accessed 2 March 2014].

Nursing and Midwifery Council (NMC) (2004) *Standards for the Preparation of Teachers of Nurses, Midwives and Specialist Community Public Health Nurses*. London: NMC.

Nursing and Midwifery Council (NMC) (2006) *Standards to Support Learning and Assessment in Practice: NMC standards for mentors, practice teachers and teachers*. London: NMC.

Nursing and Midwifery Council (NMC) (2007) *Ensuring Continuity of Practice Assessment through the Ongoing Achievement Record*, Circular 33/2007. London: NMC.

Nursing and Midwifery Council (NMC) (2008) *Standards to Support Learning and Assessment in Practice: NMC standards for mentors, practice teachers and teachers*, 2nd edn. London: NMC.

Nursing and Midwifery Council (NMC) (2010) *Standards for Pre-registration Nursing Education*. London: NMC. Available at: http://standards.nmc-uk.org/Published Documents/Standards%20for%20pre-registration%20nursing%20education%2016082010.pdf [accessed 2 March 2014].

Pulsford, D., Boit, K. and Owen, S. (2002) Are mentors ready to make a difference? A survey of mentors' attitudes towards nurse education, *Nurse Education Today*, 22(6): 439–46.

Robinson, S., Cornish, J., Driscoll, C., Knutton, S., Corben, V. and Stevenson, T. (2012) *Sustaining and Managing the Delivery of Student Nurse Mentorship: Roles, resources, standards and debates – short report*, an NHS London 'Readiness for Work' project. London: National Nursing Research Unit, King's College London.

UKCC (1999) *Fitness for Practice*. London: UK Central Council for Nursing, Midwifery and Health Visiting.

2 The effective mentor

Key points

- There are many aspects to the role of the mentor
- A student's welcome and induction is crucial in setting the tone for the placement
- Active listening is a key skill in forming effective working relationships
- Leadership and managerial skills are key aspects of mentorship
- The concept of toxic mentoring is a useful guide as to how not to do it!

NMC (2008) domains and outcomes for a mentor related to this chapter

Establish effective working relationships

- Demonstrate an understanding of factors that influence how students integrate into practice
- Provide ongoing and constructive support to facilitate transition from one learning environment to another
- Have effective professional and interprofessional working relationships to support learning for entry to the register

Create an environment for learning

- Act as a resource to facilitate the personal and professional developments of others

Context of practice

- Set and maintain professional boundaries that are sufficiently flexible for providing interprofessional care

(continued)

Evidence-based practice

- Identify and apply research- and evidence-based practice to their area of practice

Leadership

- Be an advocate for students to support them accessing learning opportunities that meet their individual needs – involving a range of other professionals, patients, clients, and carers

- Prioritise work to accommodate support of students within their practice roles

Motivation, Maslow, and mentors

The motivational theory of Abraham Maslow (1987) is described later in Chapter 4 in relation to learning and teaching theory. However, it is useful here to look at it from the practical point of view of a student on placement. In identifying an order in which we usually meet basic human needs, Maslow gives us a clue as to how to appreciate and account for the needs of our students. According to Maslow, some higher-order needs cannot be met until certain lower-order needs have been met. Physiological needs must be met first followed by the needs for security and safety, belonging, self-esteem, and finally self-actualisation. Because of this, we also need to see students as people who have lives, and therefore other needs, outside of nursing.

Physiological needs

Students will not be able to get the best out of their placement if they are not eating enough and it should be recognised that some students live within limited means. Most universities will have student hardship funds and support mechanisms for financial needs, and the mentor can involve the link tutor to help the student explore these. The student may also have problems with accommodation, or lack of sleep due to stress and the pressure of study; indeed, many students balance their full-time nursing course with paid work elsewhere. Add to this mix a 'healthy!' social life and it is easy to see why a student might be too tired to get the most out of the experiences the placement provides. A number of students will, of course, invert Maslow's hierarchy, with the need to 'belong' and 'party' taking precedence over the basics such as eating. Mentors may need to remind students about their professional responsibilities. Similarly, many students are mature and have family responsibilities. Mentors need to take account of these human stresses and strains and be realistic in their expectations and supportive, but also be assertive and offer guidance where a student is consistently falling short of expectations. An open and frank discussion should ensue and a way forward be agreed. The student can be pointed in the direction of other support mechanisms if appropriate, and the mentor may also involve the university link tutor should it become necessary.

Security and belonging needs

The need to feel secure on placement can be met by reducing anxieties, especially early on in a placement. A good orientation programme will do this with the student being met and seen early on by their mentor and inducted and introduced to others within the team. It is also important for students to feel well supported when they are asked to perform tasks with which they are unfamiliar or which are particularly demanding. By being aware of the student's level and ability, the mentor will ensure the student is adequately supported and their anxieties addressed. It also helps if students are not alone on placement but have peers they can chat to and work with. Sometimes on short placements it can be difficult to achieve a real sense of belonging, but a good mentor can help to make a student feel they are valued and can make a useful contribution, by giving them time, seeking their opinion, and making sure they are involved.

Self-esteem

This need will be met if the above ones have been met because the student will have a sense of being involved, valued, wanted, and of making a positive contribution. Being given frequent positive feedback and being included in the social as well as the working life of the clinical team will foster this even more.

Self-actualisation

Self-actualisation is a vague concept and often ill defined. Self-actualisation has been described as the achievement of ambitions and goals in professional or personal life. Others describe it as fulfilling one's potential. It is difficult for a mentor to promise this but for many students the road to this goal can be via the personal and professional achievements made on the journey through a successful placement and nurse training.

The many roles of the mentor

According to Homer's *Odyssey* (circa 800 BC), Mentor was the name of the person Odysseus asked to look after his son while he was away. The word 'mentor' now means a guardian, advisor, teacher.

According to the NMC (2006), the main responsibilities of nursing mentors include:

- Organising and coordinating student learning activities in practice
- Supervising students in learning situations
- Providing constructive feedback
- Setting and monitoring objectives
- Assessing students' skills, attitudes, and behaviours
- Providing evidence of student achievement
- Liaising with others about student performance
- Identifying concerns
- Agreeing action about concerns

Gopee (2008), among others, cites the work of Darling (1984), who suggests the following additional roles and characteristics of a mentor:

- **Role model**   Always under scrutiny and always upholding high standards and professionalism. Well respected by their peers and who the student 'looks up to' and holds in high regard. This is a powerful position of influence.

- **Energiser**   Motivating, inspiring, and enthusiastic. Seeks to use every situation as an opportunity to teach.

- **Envisioner**   Keen to embrace change and improve care, and to encourage the student to see beyond the present and seek improvements in care.

- **Investor**   Gives freely of their time, knowledge, and experience. Delegates responsibility to the student.

- **Supporter**   Available and willing to listen; encouraging. Humanistic and empathic in approach. Takes account of the student's anxieties and needs.

- **Standard prodder**   Questioning, seeking to improve standards. Demonstrates up-to-date knowledge. Matches student tasks to their level.

- **Teacher–coach**   Passes on skills and competence, guides, sets up learning experiences, allows time for practice. Encourages personal and professional development. Provides and organises a range of learning opportunities. Willing to share knowledge.

- **Feedback giver**   Gives constructive feedback, identifies future learning. Skilled questioner and facilitator of reflection. Assessor.

- **Eye opener**   Shows student the wider picture beyond the team, e.g. politics, management, research.

- **Door opener**   Points out and brokers other learning opportunities and resources, such as the wider multidisciplinary team.

- **Ideas bouncer**   Helps student reflect and generate new ideas, open to discussion and exploration of the literature.

- **Problem solver**   Helps student develop problem-solving skills. Supportive when a student is struggling.

- **Career counsellor**   Gives guidance upon future directions and possibilities.

- **Challenger**   Helps student develop critically and encourages them to question and challenge views and prevailing norms.

Other desirable qualities of a mentor include:

Assertive	Knowledgeable
Confident	Competent
Approachable	Honest
Empathic	A good listener
Experienced	Trustworthy
Patient	Accessible
Creative	Kind
Consistent	Fair
Non-judgemental	Respected by peers

The list of qualities is endless and a good mentor is many different things to many different people, but from the above list it is clear that a mentor is a dedicated professional with a real desire to further the profession of nursing by giving their time and energy to passing on their knowledge, skills, attitude, and intuition to others.

Trainee mentor describing the diversity of their role

I hadn't realised until I actually sat and watched a mentor and worked with them just exactly what it entailed. From the welcoming and inducting of the student, identifying their needs, setting up learning experiences, action planning, setting aside time to discuss things with them, assessing them and a whole lot more besides.

Effective working relationships

The foundation for being a good mentor is in building a good working relationship with the student. Achieving this one initial, important goal will solidly underpin every other aspect of mentorship and do much to reduce the usual anxieties of the student on a new placement. The contemporary scenario of the busy mentor in a short-staffed clinical area trying to balance the needs of patients, managers, and others with those of a student means that time is at a premium. As such, any time spent with the student must be very well used. For this to be the case, it is imperative that good working relationships are achieved as quickly as possible. There are two major facets to this: the first is managing the student's first day and week in a productive and welcoming way; the second is the mentor's use of good communication skills and 'active listening'.

Increased anxiety reduces learning (Moscaritolo 2009)

Why is this quote important?

Pre-placement visits

Both the student and the clinical placement staff should be aware of who is going where before the placement starts. A good student will contact the clinical team in advance of the placement to check what time they should turn up, and whether there is any uniform policy or other protocols they should be aware of. Similarly, a good ward team and mentor will encourage the student to make a preliminary visit just to be given the above information and to say 'hello'. It can help enormously to reduce anxiety on a first day if the student already knows one or two faces. The clinical team should allocate the mentor well in advance of the student arriving, and the mentor should be allocated on the basis that they can stay with the student for the duration of the placement. On a pre-placement visit, the student can be introduced to their mentor and have a quick chat and any placement reading can be handed out together with the placement information pack, outlining learning opportunities and ward information, shift pattern, dress code, and so on. Off-duty rotas can be planned together and a pre-placement visit can also be the forum for any negotiation over study days and childcare needs for example, so that the anxiety over these can be managed prior to the placement. A good welcoming pre-placement visit can begin the process of socialisation into the team and its culture and can give the student an early sense of belonging.

Pre-placement pack

Often given out prior to a student beginning a placement, this pack will include much of the material included in the induction. If you don't

(continued)

already have a pre-placement protocol and student pack, consider what should be included in one. Think back to your own experiences in the early days of placements and generate a list of useful information and things that could be achieved on such a visit. These are discussed in more detail in Chapter 3.

Student quotes

A common feature of student feedback is that of their mentor going on holiday shortly after they have begun the placement. These kinds of eventualities can easily be foreseen and thus avoided with effective pre-planning.

Third-year mental health field student on mental health adolescent unit

Although my mentor was supportive and knowledgeable, she was on annual leave for the crucial first 2 weeks of the placement, then she had further holidays and spent much of the time on nights. I felt quite isolated.

First-year adult field student on first placement (acute admissions)

I arranged and visited the unit prior to commencement of the placement. This helped to alleviate uncertainties into what awaits you and helps in building relationships prior to the dreaded 'first day at work' feeling. On the starting day, I was one hour late due to unforeseen circumstances, then I got asked by the nurse, 'What are you doing here?' My mentor was unaware that he was mentoring me and due to his holiday arrangements and night shifts I only saw him for 3 days over the next 5 weeks.

The first day and week

Newly qualified mentor

Looking back on my own placements, I can remember how nerve-wracking it is when you start a new placement. Being made to feel welcome made all the difference. I make sure that all the students are greeted with a smile – it sets the tone for the entire placement.

The important elements of the first week are building up a rapport with the student, orientation and induction to the placement, and the all-important first interview.

Building rapport

Many of the mentor attributes discussed above are the key qualities of a humanistic approach to teaching in the tradition of Carl Rogers (1994). Rogers felt that providing an appropriate culture or environment would in itself facilitate and nurture learning. A key element of this approach is developing a relationship with the student which is respectful of their autonomy and in which the mentor displays the qualities of genuineness, respect, trust, acceptance, and empathy. According to Rogers, genuineness is about being your real self rather than presenting with a false role or pretending to be some sort of ideal type. An effective mentor does not pretend to be perfect or that they know all the answers. They are real people who are still learning themselves but are willing to share what they do know. Good mentors are non-judgemental about their students, and thus are able to develop a relationship based upon trust and acceptance. Only in such an open and trusting atmosphere can a student really feel at ease and free to ask for help and to question.

Stupid question?

One sign of a good learning environment and good mentor is that the student feels able to ask any question no matter how 'silly' it might seem, without fear of being shot down and ridiculed.

There is no such thing as a stupid question, just learning opportunities.

Within such a relationship, the student will feel respected rather than awkward and incompetent. This is especially important in the early stages of training where many students will be both young and inexperienced in healthcare matters. The mentor needs to strip away some of the awe in which they can find themselves shrouded.

Awestruck!

A first-year student on their first placement and who has no previous healthcare experience is looking quite scared after shadowing you for the morning. Close to tears, they tell you they don't think they can do it, that they'll never get to be as skilled and professional as you.

What would you say to this student?

Having insight into the student's needs will allow the mentor to display a degree of empathic understanding, which will make the student feel more at ease. A bit of self-disclosure on the mentor's part can go a long way here, reassuring the student that they were once a novice and that the student will also become competent. Such empathy can do much for developing the student's confidence that they, too, will achieve the same professionalism and standard as their mentor.

Displaying and using Rogers' core conditions as described above will allow you to build a relationship with the student in which each other's expectations can be shared in a trusting and open way.

First-year adult nursing student on mental health placement

I was really quite apprehensive and it must have shown because my mentor took me to a quiet room and we sat and had a chat about the ward and what to expect. She just sat and listened, but more importantly took me seriously.

Consistency on the part of the mentor is also important in building trust. The mentor must do what they say they will and not embark upon a pattern of excuses for not having time and postponing agreed meetings. In many respects, finding the time is the hardest part of mentoring but it is crucial to do so.

Taking the student as they are is also important and this means that the mentor must be non-judgemental and display what Rogers calls unconditional positive regard. An effective mentor is capable of being objective and has an awareness of their own prejudices and preconceptions and will not allow themselves to be swayed by such.

Wilkes (2006) reminds us that although we should seek to bond with the student, we must keep the relationship professional. Developing too deep a social or emotional relationship will make it difficult for a mentor to act professionally, and assessments are likely to be compromised regarding validity and objectivity.

Question

What might be the underlying reasons for a student trying to cultivate a friendship rather than a professional relationship?

Welcome and orientation

Orientation is the gateway to a successful placement (Beskine 2009).

The initial welcome and orientation is a crucial phase in helping the student get off on the right foot and make the most of their placement. At the outset, it is useful to share a little of your own experiences of being a student and to talk a little about yourself, and to ask the student about their experiences so far and a little about themselves outside of nursing. Gray and Smith (2000) highlight the importance of the early days of a placement, reporting that a good orientation experience reduces the dependency of the student upon the mentor. Ensure the first shift is not too busy and that you have time to spend with the student. Gray and Smith (2000, p. 1546) cite one student from their study who made just this point, that if the first shift is a morning shift, 'you are just going to be used as a pair of hands ... Whereas if staff roster you on a back shift they are more willing to give you time for a proper orientation.' The orientation should include introducing the student to the ward team and giving them a tour of the area. Essential information should be provided, including fire and emergency procedures, location of essential equipment, and security issues.

First-year adult field student on children's ward

I was made to feel part of the team and felt well supported. The orientation day was very useful and you became prepared for what to expect from the department, they taught us some basic skills. I felt much more confident after this session.

First interview

The first interview really sets the tone of the placement and puts the student at ease. The following is a list of things that should be covered at this early stage:

- Deal with any anxieties the student may have regarding the placement. These may range from unmet objectives from previous placements to worries in relation to their ability, including concerns about the client group or type of experience. These concerns need to be listened to and dealt with early on so that the student can concentrate upon the placement.

- Clarify general information about contact details, shifts, and breaks.

- The student should be introduced to the ward/team philosophy and made aware of the location and importance of adhering to local procedures and policies.

- It is important to identify the student's level and stage of training, and clearly ascertain their learning needs. Mentors need to work closely with students in the first week to assess their level of competence and accurately gauge the level of supervision required, as the mentor remains accountable for any tasks they delegate to the student. (See Chapter 8, 'Supporting failing students', for a more in-depth discussion of the importance of this.)

- Initially, set achievable objectives so that the student can be up and running almost straight away. It will boost their confidence if they are able to achieve some objectives early on in a placement.

- Discuss the student's need to experience the full range of shifts and days.

- Ask if there is anything they need to do linked to assignments. Students can come to placements worried about assignments and it can become their prime focus if the mentor is not careful. As a link tutor, I visit students on placement wanting to discuss their placement experiences, but am often confronted with an anxious student who only want to talk about their assignments.

- Ask if there are any essential skills assessments they need to achieve within the placement. Plan the necessary practice sessions and set clear dates for the summative assessments, or for reviewing progress.

- At the initial interview, the mentor should explain to the student the clinical learning opportunities that are available and how best to access them.

- Discuss the importance of reflection and how you will facilitate this.

- Identify dates for subsequent, more formal interviews.

- Make known objectives for shifts when you cannot be with the student, and identify a named co-mentor or 'associate mentor' who will support them in your absence.

- Point out learning resources, such as internet access, books, journals, and any study area.

- Ask about their strengths and areas they would like to work on. There may be things they have been avoiding or haven't had the opportunity to do as yet. Many mental health students, for example, become quite anxious about giving an intramuscular injection, some because they don't like the idea and some because all their peers have done this and they feel that they are behind.

- Reiterate issues around professionalism and motivation, timekeeping, and confidentiality.

In general, the overall impression of the student should be one of an enthusiastic and competent mentor who will make sure they get a good experience if they themselves put the effort in. The initial interview is thus a good time to remind students of their responsibilities.

First-year student on oncology placement

Having such a good mentor enabled me to learn many new skills. From the start of the placement I felt like part of the team, and they created a great environment to learn in. They guided you towards the knowledge base.

The initial interview is also the place to discuss the student's own responsibility towards the placement and their own learning. It is important that students do not become too reliant upon the mentor and should begin learning to shoulder some responsibility early on in their training.

Student's placement responsibilities

- Contact the placement in advance and establish start time and dress code, etc.
- Undergo all induction tasks.
- Act professionally in relation to timekeeping, dress, attitude, and confidentiality.
- Identify your own learning needs.
- Take responsibility for your learning needs.
- Be honest about your ability and level of competence.
- Ask for help when unsure.
- Always respect the client's dignity and individuality.
- Actively participate and seek out learning opportunities.
- Ensure you take time to reflect.
- Identify and undertake insight visits with the wider multidisciplinary team.
- Practise good communication and a willingness to work with the team.
- Ensure placement paperwork is kept up to date.
- Present your mentor with evidence of achievement at regular intervals.
- Act upon constructive feedback.
- Ensure assessment documentation is completed and submitted.
- Evaluate and provide feedback on the placement.

Guidance on Professional Conduct for Nursing and Midwifery Students (NMC 2009)

This mirrors the checklist above and can be downloaded at www.nmcuk. org (under publications and guidance). It can form a very useful basis for discussion around the student's responsibilities.

Second-year student on surgical ward

When I raised my concerns about my lack of input from my mentor, my issues were addressed quickly. I was expecting my mentor to shepherd me all the time. Now I realise I need to just muck in and get on and seek out opportunities for myself sometimes.

Induction checklist

The clinical area should have its own induction schedule for students which they have to complete within the first couple of days and tick off and date to show they have undertaken what is necessary. Often this can be adapted from that used for new staff. There will be variations according to clinical specialty but it should include the following:

- Tour of area and facilities
- Staff introductions (key staff to meet)
- Contact information (team and student)
- Clinic times and policies regarding sickness and uniform
- Key policies and locations (e.g. clinical, health and safety, moving and handling, lone worker policies, close observation, escorting clients, Mental Health Act)
- Procedures in case of fire, call numbers, alarms, equipment, escape and assembly points
- Emergency and resuscitation procedures, equipment, and call numbers
- Location and use of moving and handling equipment
- Waste disposal, control of infection
- Prevention and management of violence, and aggression policy and procedures
- Incident reporting
- Security issues

Second-year mental health student on adult medical ward

The orientation to the ward and induction pack was great, it helped us to work through things even when staff were busy and couldn't devote the time to showing the students.

Active listening: the basis of effective working relationships

Achieving Rogers' core conditions is an important foundation for an effective relationship with the student, and good communication skills are required to make it work. Perhaps the most useful communication skill in mentoring is that of active listening. The mentor who regularly takes the time to listen to the student's concerns and frequently canvasses their opinion is laying the foundation of a good working relationship. Essentially, active listening is the ability to listen attentively, concentrating upon what the person is saying and making them aware that you are doing so. This sounds a bit simplistic, but it is easy to listen and not hear (i.e. forget half of what the person has told you). It is also easy to listen and give the other person the impression you are not interested. Both of these will quickly bring the conversation to a close and therefore be of little use. The key elements of active listening bring together a range of verbal and non-verbal skills that aim to convey your interest and develop the communication. In counselling scenarios, the active listener is trying to get the speaker to open up and describe their predicament in detail in order to help them explore it and its meaning for them. The skill is in blending the non-verbal elements such as eye contact and posture with the verbal elements such as questioning skills.

Non-verbal elements of active listening

The non-verbal elements of communication are often overlooked and taken for granted. However, they are just as important as the verbal elements in conveying to the speaker the interest and concern of the listener.

Egan (2002) summarises the non-verbal elements of communication by suggesting the acronym SOLER as a guide to helping us to 'tune in' to the other person and give them our full attention:

S   Sit squarely or slightly angled, facing the student indicating involvement

O   Open posture, no folded arms or defensive, excluding postures

L   Lean towards and orient yourself to the student to show interest

E   Eye contact, ensure it is steady and natural, not threatening

R   Relax, be comfortable, and be yourself. Try not to fidget

The following are some tips for improving non-verbal communication:

Give good eye contact

Don't stare directly at the person as this can be off-putting, uncomfortable, and be misconstrued as aggressive. The British are said to be quite reserved and not to like a great deal of eye contact. Other cultures interpret this low level of eye contact as disinterest, preferring a much more direct and prolonged gaze. This fits in with the belief that a person who will not look you in the eye has something to hide and is generally not to be trusted. Good eye contact means different things to each of us, but in general look at the person directly from time to time and keep reinforcing this contact.

Facial expression

This provides the listener with a window into the emotional state of the speaker and vice versa. We need to ensure that we pick up on subtle clues and act upon them, for example, 'you seem quite annoyed by that', or 'you look confused'. Facial expression can often let you know whether someone understands or not. Similarly, we need to ensure that our facial expressions denote our interest in the speaker and do not suggest disinterest and boredom. An occasional smile and nod of the head will often be sufficient to let the speaker know we are still with them. It is worth remembering that it is relatively easy to lie verbally but much harder to lie non-verbally.

Overcome your own concerns

You cannot listen effectively to another person if you cannot put aside your own personal issues, such as being worried about whether your car will get clamped or ruminating upon your own personal issues. You need to give the other person your complete attention.

Don't be put off by silences

Moments of silence are important in allowing the speaker to reflect upon what they have said and formulate what they wish to say next. In emotional circumstances, they can feel awkward and there is a tendency for the listener to bring silences to a premature end because they are uncomfortable; this denies the speaker the opportunity to feel and express their emotion, which is a necessary part of the process if they are to come to terms with it and explore their worries further.

Avoid distractions

Ensure that you arrange for privacy and no interruptions. Let others know that you are in a private meeting and hang a sign on the door.

Paralinguistics

Tone of voice is the obvious example here. Again, this can give us significant clues as to the emotional state of the speaker and how they feel about what they are saying. We use tone of voice to express aggression and passion, as well as a range of other emotional states. Other vocal aspects of non-verbal behaviour are the 'grunts' and similar noises we make in conversation to reaffirm we are listening. These are the 'aha' and 'mmm' sounds we make, which we use in conjunction with an often unconscious nodding of the head to demonstrate that we understand.

Posture

Sitting or leaning slightly forward towards the speaker suggests that you are interested in what they have to say, just as leaning away implies that you are not. We tend to keep a safe distance from those we are wary of and get close to those we are fond of, and this delivers a simple but powerful message. Similarly, fidgeting suggests anxiety and we should be alert to such signs in the student.

Verbal elements and questioning skills

While non-verbal skills enable you to display interest and concern in the speaker, it is the verbal skills that help you to clarify and explore the content of what is being said in order to gain a greater depth of understanding of the speaker's position. The following are some tips for improving your verbal and questioning skills:

Explore feelings

If a person is angry, sad or emotional, the listener has to help them address those feelings before they can explore any other issues. The student who is upset at a failed assessment will need to be allowed to express and explore their emotions before discussing the way forward. You can't discuss an action plan with an angry or tearful student.

Don't interrupt

Let the other person finish before you jump in with your views. It is a natural tendency to want to do this, but it is disrespectful and may cut the speaker off when working up to something they feel strongly about.

Be challenging

This is about keeping a meeting or discussion on track. Having said above 'don't interrupt', you may have to bring the dialogue back on track because it is easy to avoid a difficult situation by skirting around the issue and filling the time with unrelated material. A student might need to be prompted and guided back onto the core subject matter under discussion. There are usually good reasons as to why a person is reluctant. In *The Skilled Helper*, Egan (2002) points out that every now and again we need to be challenged to move forward. Occasionally, we become stuck for a variety of reasons; for example, we may be anxious or avoiding a situation and need to be challenged to confront that fear and work through it. We all occasionally suffer from what Egan calls the 'blind spots' of unawareness, self-deception, choosing to stay in the dark, or knowing but not caring. Only when these are challenged and acknowledged can the person work on them and move on.

Self-disclosure

A little self-disclosure can go a long way towards letting the speaker appreciate you have similar experiences and know how they might feel. However, make sure you don't hijack the conversation and lose the focus upon the student. In counselling sessions, a client may try to get the counsellor to speak about their life because it deflects attention away from themselves and the difficult task of dealing with their own problems.

Summarise

You can't possibly remember everything, so occasionally, at appropriate points, stop the conversation and summarise what you understand the person has been saying. This will allow you to make sure you have got it right and understood correctly. If you are wrong, the student will tell you and clarify the situation. It also tells the student that you have been listening to them and so encourages further dialogue.

Open questions

'What do you think should have been done?' and 'How did you feel when you . . . ?' are questions that demand more than a 'yes' or 'no' answer and lead the speaker to divulge further information. They try to get the person to open up and explore the subject in greater depth. Try not to use closed questions or leading questions, as these will stifle the conversation and lead to an incomplete, unshared or biased view.

Try to turn the following closed questions into open ones:

Do you think that is the best way to do it?

Would you do it the same way again?

Will you be able to manage?

Did you manage to do it?

Should that go there?

Clarifying questions

'What did you say you did when that happened . . . ?' and 'What do you mean when you say . . . ?' are examples of questions that will help you make sure you have got the story right and help avoid any ambiguity.

Probing questions

The following questions let you delve deeper and help to clarify the position: 'Can you tell me a bit more about that?', 'What does that mean in terms of your future learning needs?', 'Why do you think it could have been prevented?', 'Why is that important?'.

Hypothetical questions

The following questions will help the student to think more creatively and elevate their learning from experience to a higher level: 'What do you think would happen if . . . ?', 'What else would you have to do if . . . ?', 'If money was no object, how would you improve . . . ?'.

Reflection

This entails occasionally reflecting back to the speaker in order to clarify your understanding of what has been said. It can also demonstrate that you were listening carefully. You can do this by 'echoing' back what the person has said exactly as they said it, or you can 'paraphrase' it by putting it into your own words. The person will either say 'Yes, that's right . . . ' or 'No, that's not how I see it, what I meant was . . . '. Either way, you have clarified your understanding of the situation and they have been reassured that you want to get it right and are listening attentively.

Non-verbal exercises

As a lesson in self-awareness, arrange with a colleague to record on DVD an interview conducted by the two of you. Equipment can usually be borrowed from the School of Nursing. Take turns to be interviewed and to interview, discussing some work-related issue. The interviewer's job is to draw out the information from the interviewee. Try to summarise occasionally and clarify where necessary. When you have finished, watch the recording together and discuss the skills used by the interviewer. Take note of your non-verbal behaviour and identify and discuss the questioning techniques used. This is a good exercise in practising these skills and also an opportunity to see how we come across to others both visually and behaviourally, as we are often unaware of our non-verbal 'habits'.

Evidence-based practice

An effective mentor will be more effective if they have the capability of using evidence-based practice. A student witnessing a mentor researching the evidence for a procedure and altering their practice by applying that evidence, will gain an impression of nursing as a dynamic and

(continued)

forward-thinking profession as opposed to one that routinely and blindly accepts current practice and routine as the norm. A mentor can also demonstrate this by attendance at training sessions, workshops, and conferences. They might also ensure the ward has access to current journals of relevance to the specialty and by directing the students to such. Fostering an enquiring spirit in students can also be achieved by asking the student to seek out information and relay this back to the team. Another important aspect of evidence-based practice is the mentor's use of it to underpin their mentoring. The material discussed above is all evidence-based, as are teaching skills and it is important that the mentor understands the theory behind different styles of learning in order to teach effectively. In effect, they are applying research- and evidence-based practice to their mentoring.

Student-centred leadership

To be an effective mentor, certain leadership skills are useful. The Leadership domain highlights:

- Being organised, so that you can effectively plan learning experiences that meet the students' individual needs

- Advocating on behalf of students to help them access multidisciplinary learning opportunities

- Prioritising practice work and managing your time to ensure you can provide support to students

- Providing feedback about the effectiveness of the clinical learning experience

It is often hard to describe exactly what these management skills are but key indicators and leadership traits from the NHS KSF Leadership dimension hold strong resonance for mentors here. These include:

- Ensuring individuals meet their goals and have been given clear expectations of performance

- People feel well led and 'heard'

- People get clear feedback

- Client (student) focused

- Develops individual people and teamwork ethos

- Develops an open, questioning, and supportive culture

- Having self-belief

- Being prepared to face challenges
- Effective decision-making
- Prepared to be accountable and hold people to account
- Role models ethical behaviour and champions values and standards

A mentor displaying these qualities will ensure that students know what is expected of them and they will feel well supported. They will believe they are getting a planned, well thought through, and challenging placement experience that will develop their potential.

Management skills such as those outlined above will also play a large part in helping to foster a student-centred culture in a clinical area.

Exercise

Imagine you have just gained promotion to team leader. Student feedback and anecdotal evidence tell you that the clinical team has a history of negativity towards students and being used as a placement. Some staff feel they are too specialist and too busy and one or two staff members are, to put it bluntly, lazy when it comes to the idea of supporting students. Several also have a distinct disdain for 'modern' nurse training.

As the 'new' manager, write an action plan for trying to turn this situation around and list the benefits for the whole team of becoming a student-friendly environment.

Toxic mentoring (how not to do it!)

An examination of how not to do something is usually a good guide to how to do it well by identifying negative behaviours that should be avoided. The concept of 'toxic mentoring' describes those behaviours.

A student experience

They were never there. Even on the days we were rostered to work the same shifts he was either off doing something else or he'd changed shifts. I ended up working with anyone who'd have me, or just doing stuff off my own bat. When we did work together he just gave me menial stuff to do, and when I did get to do something more interesting he never asked me about it or told me I'd done well. I think we only worked with each other about 8 times and yet he signed all my paperwork! I didn't learn much but I passed!

In a busy clinical area where there are huge demands on the mentor's time, and some mentors for various reasons do not particularly like mentoring students, various behaviours have a negative impact upon the student experience and have come to be known collectively as 'toxic mentoring'.

How not to do it

If you were a 'toxic' mentor, list the ways in which you could sabotage and detract from a student's learning experience.

The impact of toxic mentoring can be devastating for students, as evidenced by the following quotes:

Quotations from student placement feedback

Student midwife

It really shocked me that she had assigned herself to work with students and should be an inspiration to them. I left the shift completely disillusioned.

First-year adult nurse

The first encounter with my mentor was at the beginning of my second week on the ward, and this was an experience I shall never forget. She was rude and aggressive towards me and I didn't want to go in the next day.

Mental health student on adult placement

There were many procedures done on a daily basis, but we were never asked to watch or help.

Adult nurse student on adult ward acute placement

The placement would have been a lot better if my mentor found things for me to do instead of leaving me alone. It made me feel very useless.

Mental health student on adult placement

She did my final interview without me. When I went in, in my own time, she said she couldn't be bothered to do it and would do it at home later.

Second-year adult nurse student

I spent an awful lot of time just hanging around. It would be nice to have a mentor to work with and not one who spends all the time in the office.

(continued)

Adult field student on mental health placement

Because of me being an adult field student, the mental health field student got more of a look in than me because it was her intended field.

Adult student on adult placement

Basically, I spent the days making beds and working with the care assistants.

Second-year mental health student on child and adolescent mental health placement

Because of the challenges presented when working with young people and the emotions invoked from doing so, effective mentorship is essential. I often felt that the mentor dismissed my concerns, especially around restraint, as they were so familiar with the environment. Mentorship and supervision is essential here, especially in the first few weeks of a placement and needs to be formal and regular.

Mentor to adult student on theatre placement

There's no point in teaching you anything, you're only here for a fortnight.

Adult field student on accident and emergency placement

My final interview consisted of my mentor criticising my outcome evidence. She gave me no verbal praise or feedback and her comments were written without discussion. I didn't feel I could approach her to discuss the issue, as over the course of my placement my confidence had been somewhat undermined.

Adult field student on being asked how the placement could have been improved

A different mentor.

Third-year adult field student

If my mentor had given me more tasks to perform and more responsibility, it would have been OK. As a third year I am supposed to be nearly competent and need to develop my nursing skills but I wasn't given much chance.

Davies et al. (1994) found that mentors gave structure, planning, and meaning to the students' learning experience compared with students who had no mentor, who felt they were left largely just 'hanging about' purposelessly trying to slot in somewhere and make the best of it. Such a feeling is common to students who experience toxic mentoring.

Darling (1986) identifies four broad types of toxic mentor and others have identified variants on the same theme:

- **Avoiders.** Avoiders simply are never available for a variety of reasons. This can lead to the student not being able to key into the placement and the team, and so not being able to fully exploit all the placement has to offer. It is a simple strategy for mentors to arrange and stick to meetings with the student and there is no real excuse for not doing so. Occasionally, the realistic excuse of being too busy will hold water but the regular occurrence of this phenomenon indicates a mentor who is not at all committed to the task.

- **Dumpers.** These mentors put students into difficult situations and give them tasks well out of their depth and offer no assistance. This can obviously be dangerous and can have a devastating impact upon a student's confidence. Such a student will be very unlikely to ask the mentor for anything else to do and is likely to spend the rest of the placement with their head well down trying to avoid the mentor. This type of mentor will also take little responsibility for organising meetings or learning experiences, leaving it all up to the student. This is an abdication of responsibility. Such mentors are also likely to 'dump' unwanted jobs upon the student.

- **Blockers.** Such mentors actively refuse students' requests for help or experience and withhold information, or over-supervise the student thus limiting their development.

- **Destroyers/criticisers.** These mentors damage students' self-esteem by being negative and concentrating on faults rather than strengths. At its worst this is done in public and has a marked impact on students' confidence. Such mentors tend to have an over-inflated view of their own competence and can regard themselves as experts. Such a level of arrogance can be very off-putting for the novice student. One of the prime joys of being a mentor should be in embracing the challenge which students present. The welcoming of questioning minds and the desire to find out from the student any new theories or updates learnt in the university is a bonus. Once this desire is lost, the mentor needs to reconsider their role.

List of toxic mentor behaviours

- Works with student much less than 40% of the time

- Frequently cancels meetings

- Regards student as a care assistant

- Does not let student do anything unsupervised

- Does not take account of level of learner

- Does not find out students' learning needs

(continued)

- Puts students in difficult unsupervised positions
- Does not broker learning experiences
- Frequently asks others to 'look after' the student
- Leaves the student to arrange everything themselves
- Does not engage student in reflection on experience
- Feedback focuses on deficits and 'weaknesses'
- Does not help with action plans
- Takes no responsibility for student learning
- Does not attend mentor updates
- Is unfamiliar with the student's paperwork and assessment
- Rarely aware of the evidence behind their own practice
- Does not acknowledge students' prior experience
- Reluctant to embrace change
- Displays unprofessional behaviour
- Does not work well with the multidisciplinary team

Supernumerary status

A common feature of toxic mentoring is the convenient forgetting of the supernumerary status of the student, who immediately becomes an extra pair of hands and is rostered as an extra healthcare assistant. To a team manager on a budget, this represents a saving in not having to 'buy' in bank staff, but essentially this is an abuse of the student's learning needs. Students are additional to the usual workforce requirements.

Third-year student on medical ward

I was finally given a mentor in week 4 and I was given my next shifts. I assumed they would be the same as my mentor's but they were actually the opposite shifts to his. When I asked if I could change my shifts, the deputy sister said 'no', as I had been given the shifts as they were short-staffed on those days and if I swapped there would be a staff shortage. During the whole placement I felt like I was being used to cover a shortfall in staff. If the senior staff saw me they would take away the healthcare assistant and say they were not needed, as there was a student there.

(continued)

Second-year mental health field student on mental health admission ward

More support should have been given to the students by the staff but also more support given to the mentors. When I first arrived on the ward, no one knew who I was and they said they were not expecting me. Also, no one knew who my mentor was and it took them a while to allocate me a mentor. They seemed unorganised for students.

The NMC dictates that all student experiences should be 'educationally led'. However, this is not to say that the student should not 'muck in' and perform the day-to-day tasks common to busy clinical areas. In general, the advice that 'you get out of it what you put into it' holds true for placements. There is much to be gleaned from 'buddying' with a healthcare support worker and drawing upon their years of experience. This is a vital part of the student's learning experience, but not the mainstay of it. Mentors and teams who do not utilise their healthcare support workers should consider the benefits of doing so for all concerned. Formalising this 'buddy' role can greatly enhance the status and self-esteem of the healthcare support workers we often take for granted. This is explored in greater depth in Chapter 9.

How can a student deal effectively with a toxic mentor?

Darling, who first coined the term 'toxic mentor', suggests that students build a support network of others whom they can turn to, but this is easier said than done and does little to help the 'stranded' student (Darling 1986). Such students are unfortunate and it takes a degree of assertiveness and courage for a student to speak out. Some students 'cope' by avoiding their mentor by working different shifts. Often the student will have the support of their peers and fellow students on the ward and they will try to access other 'associate' mentors and staff in order to try and salvage their placement experience. This is not always possible and the student should try to be assertive and request a meeting with their mentor. At this meeting they should point out what it is they feel aggrieved about and what they would like from the mentor. If necessary, they could seek support and request the presence of their university link tutor who would act as their advocate if necessary. Should things not improve, the student should request a new mentor. It is always difficult for students to undergo what ostensibly is the process of complaining, as there is a natural tendency to fear that they will not pass the placement if they 'upset' their mentor. However, students have a responsibility to themselves and to the students who follow them to ensure they get a good learning experience. Ultimately, if this is not happening after meetings have been held, then the student should be encouraged and supported in filing a formal complaint. The 'toxic' mentor is in breach of both their employment

(continued)

contract and, as Quinn and Hughes (2007) point out, their professional code of conduct. The student needs to keep a clear account of deficits and negative behaviours so that they have an accurate and objective record upon which to base their claims.

There is much anecdotal evidence that student complaints about their placements only surface in post-placement evaluations for the reasons hinted at above: they have left (and hopefully passed) the placement and need not face the person concerned again. Much of the onus here lies with the universities and schools of nursing in ensuring that they have in place good student support mechanisms and that students feel that they will be supported if they have worries and concerns and need to access that support.

From the student learning perspective, actually dealing with the problem and if necessary pursuing a complaint will be a 'good' learning experience of how to deal with negative staff for whom they will have responsibility once qualified.

The university will have in place a placement evaluation mechanism whereby such negative experiences of students will be followed up and explored and if necessary appropriate action taken. Such action might be a refresher mentor course, buddying a more experienced mentor or a disciplinary action by the employer.

Mentor SWOT analysis

A SWOT (Strengths, Weaknesses, Opportunities, Threats) analysis is a simple and effective way of examining your own mentorship role and helping you develop and improve it. This is an extremely efficient method of reflection that will help you to explore your practice in detail and often highlights issues hitherto not apparent:

- Strengths are your positive attributes and resources that enhance your ability to mentor a student.

- Weaknesses are aspects you feel you need to improve upon or skills you lack, aspects that you feel detract from your ability to be a good mentor.

- Opportunities are the resources and opportunities you have around you which you might be able to access and which support you in the role.

- Threats are the pressures and practicalities and other aspects of your role and responsibilities that might get in the way and hamper your ability to be a good mentor.

Use the SWOT analysis to list your own personal qualities and strengths, and examine the weaknesses and threats to your role as a mentor.

The following amalgamation of several SWOT analyses from nurses on a mentorship course gives some idea of the positives and negatives they recorded:

Strengths	Weaknesses
Communication skills	Lack of experience as a mentor
Work well in a team	Find it hard to delegate, 'need to be in control'
Sound knowledge base	
Experienced	Unsure about teaching skills
Timekeeping	Don't know much about curriculum
Organised	Little leadership experience
Willingness to teach	Not sure about the paperwork
Professional	Lack of confidence about assessment
Motivated	
Non-judgemental	Nervous about giving criticism
Sense of humour	Find it hard to fail someone
Fair	Poor time management
Love my job	Tend to leave things to the last minute
Accessible	
Supportive	

Opportunities	Threats
Many students in area	Pressurised ward/heavy caseload
Plenty of opportunity to be an associate mentor	Time constraints, not being able to give the students enough time
Doing the mentor course	
Good university link tutor	Staff shortages
Good peer support	Stressful environment at times
Clinic is good learning environment	No other mentors on ward
Many skills I could teach	Little support from other staff
Existing mentors to get help and learn from	
Many opportunities to work with other disciplines and specialist nurses	

Merely identifying your strengths, weaknesses, opportunities, and threats can lead to useful insights, but the real value of the analysis is when it is used to identify personal development goals. These goals will be centred on consolidating strengths and thinking about how best you can use them. The goals will also be about eradicating or overcoming weaknesses, exploiting opportunities, and nullifying threats. Such goals should then become the focus of an action plan in order to take advantage of the insights gained. Try to set time limits to your action plan and ensure that your objectives are SMART (i.e. Small, Measurable, Achievable, Realistic, Timed).

The following are just a few of the goals and ideas derived from nurses undertaking a mentor course:

Goal	Action
Become more aware of student outcomes	Try mapping the outcomes to the clinic's learning opportunities
Gain confidence in assessment	Co-assess with a current mentor and sit in on assessments
Adapt teaching and learning opportunity to level of student	Work with associate mentor as much as possible, identify level of current students and identify appropriate tasks
Become familiar with the paperwork	Ask current student to explain theirs to me, check with link tutor
Practise teaching skills	Do teaching sessions for current students and healthcare support workers
Find out more about curriculum	Ask link tutor
Qualify as a mentor	Complete the mentor course
Ensure time will be available	Speak with manager regarding expectations and time for students

A useful alternative

Another excellent way to use this tool is to ask a student you are mentoring to do a SWOT analysis of their experience of your mentoring. The benefit of this is that it is not your opinion about yourself but a more objective outside view. It is helpful because we often see things differently from each other, and are often unaware of how we come across to other people, so it is good to get another opinion to contrast with our own. When you hear a tape recording of your own voice, you may be taken aback at how different you sound, but that is how other people hear you. The student's SWOT analysis of you will let you know how you come across to them.

Liaison with higher education institutions

To be an effective mentor, you need the support of your partner in training, the higher education institution (HEI), university or School of Nursing. Good links here can make both the student's and mentor's life much easier. It is the HEI's role to support both the students and the mentors usually via a named link tutor or some other form of practice learning support. Such a link tutor will be able to help mentors keep abreast of changes to the course structure and paperwork, and be there to advise new mentors and advise on creating a good learning environment. The link tutor can also help mentors to map placement learning opportunities to the competencies students must meet and with interpreting those competencies for specific clinical areas. The HEI will usually also provide the local mentor training programme and provide regular mentor updates.

The student's personal tutor will also be a source of support. They will keep an eye on the student's progress throughout their training and can be supportive in forming action plans where concerns are raised with particular students.

Questions that might be considered useful in relation to your own clinical area

- What links do you have with the university?
- Who is your named link person?
- How can you extend the link?
- What information does the university give you prior to placing students?
- What other information would you like?
- What involvement (teaching) could you have within the university?
- What feedback about the placement do you get and can this be improved upon?
- Do you know how to access a student's personal tutor?
- Do you know how to access mentor updates?
- Is there a protocol for dealing with difficult situations?

It is a good idea to explore the ways in which mentors and the ward team can become more involved within the School of Nursing or university by, for example, undertaking teaching sessions and giving good practice workshops. Similarly, it is worthwhile investing some time in thinking about ways in which you can exploit the expertise within the university and create stronger links with the ward. This is discussed in Chapter 3, 'The clinical learning environment'.

Qualities of a mentor

As part of mentorship training on the last day of the course, students are asked to reflect upon their own student experiences and experiences of co-mentoring students and to come up with 'Ten golden rules for mentors'. These in general reflect the qualities that are most highly regarded by students and fellow mentors. An example of one such is reproduced here.

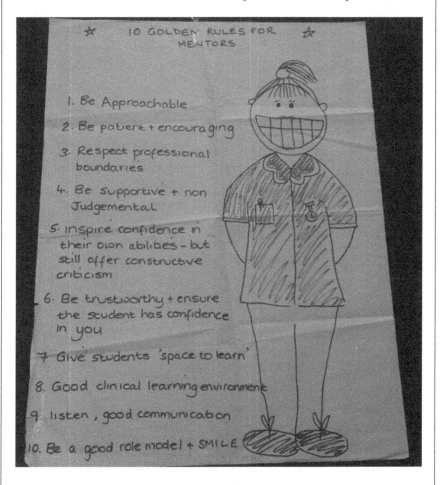

Other posters included the following advice:

Being able to remember when they were a student

Being a good leader/manager

Being organised

Setting initial expectations early on

(continued)

Flexibility	Setting a good example (role model)
Firm, fair, and consistent	Having a good relationship with university staff
Being able to challenge students	Resourceful
Enthusiastic	Knowledgeable (evidence-based)
Willing to teach	Confident
Open-minded	Reflective
Having a sense of humour	See student as an individual
Familiar with paperwork	Creates/plans learning experiences
Recognises student's level	Making time
Maintains professional boundaries	Deals with 'issues' early on
Enjoys what they are doing	And always having a good supply of biscuits!

Summary

This chapter has:

- Looked at the diversity of the role of the mentor
- Highlighted the importance of a good working relationship and the interpersonal skills which foster this
- Assessed the qualities of an effective mentor
- Described how to facilitate the initial stages of the student's placement
- Identified how 'toxic' mentors can sabotage a placement experience and what students can do if they encounter such a toxic mentor
- Described the use of a SWOT analysis to enable mentors to audit their mentoring skills and produce a personal development plan

The next chapter examines the mentor's clinical area and what it takes to make it a positive learning environment.

Further reading

Agnew, T. (2005) Words of wisdom, *Nursing Standard*, 20(6): 24–6. This is a useful look at the relationship between students and mentors.

Ali, P.A. and Panther, W. (2008) Professional development and the role of mentorship, *Nursing Standard*, 22(42): 35–9.

Andrews, M. and Chilton, F. (2000) Student and mentor perceptions of mentoring effectiveness, *Nurse Education Today*, 20(7): 555–62.

Andrews, M. and Wallis, M. (1999) Mentorship in nursing: a literature review, *Journal of Advanced Nursing*, 29(1): 201–7.

Bennett, C.L. (2003) How to be a good mentor, *Nursing Standard*, 17(36): 1–14.

Hodges, B. (2009) Factors that can influence mentorship relationships, *Paediatric Nursing*, 21(6): 32–5.

Loffmark, A. and Wikbla, K. (2001) Facilitating and obstructing factors for development of learning in clinical practice: a student nurse perspective, *Journal of Advanced Nursing*, 43(1): 43–50.

Musinski, B. (1999) The educator as facilitator: a new kind of leadership, *Nursing Forum*, 34(1): 23–9. This article reiterates much of what we have said, in that it is increasingly recognised that the participation of the learner is vital for effective education to occur. The mentor should act as facilitator, creating an environment conducive to learning that motivates individuals to want to learn.

Price, B. (2003) Mentoring learners in practice. Number 6. Building a rapport with the learner, *Nursing Standard*, 19(22): 1–2.

Raine, R. (2005) I'm sorry, what did you say your name was again?, *Mental Health Practice*, 8(10): 40–4.

Royal College of Nursing (RCN) (2002) *Helping Students Get the Best from Their Practice Placements: A Royal College of Nursing toolkit*. London: RCN.

References

Beskine, D. (2009) Mentoring students: establishing effective working relationships, *Nursing Standard*, 23(30): 35–40.

Darling, L.A.W. (1984) What do nurses want in a mentor?, *Journal of Nursing Administration*, 14(10): 42–4.

Darling, L.A.W. (1986) What to do about toxic mentors, *Nurse Educator*, 11(2): 42–4.

Davies, B., Neary, M. and Phillips, R. (1994) *The Practitioner-Teacher: A study in the introduction of mentors in the Preregistration Nurse Education Programme in Wales*. Cardiff: School of Education, University of Cardiff.

Egan, G. (2002) *The Skilled Helper: A problem management and opportunity development approach to helping*, 7th edn. Pacific Grove, CA: Brooks/Cole.

Gopee, N. (2008) *Mentoring and Supervision in Healthcare*. London: Sage.

Gray, M.A. and Smith, L.N. (2000) The qualities of an effective mentor from the student nurse's perspective: findings from a longitudinal study, *Journal of Advanced Nursing*, 32(6): 1542–9.

Maslow, A. (1987) *Motivation and Personality*, 3rd edn. New York: Harper & Row.

Moscaritolo, L.M. (2009) Interventional strategies to decrease nursing student anxiety in the clinical learning environment, *Journal of Nursing Education*, 48(1): 17–23.

Nursing and Midwifery Council (NMC) (2006) *Standards to Support Learning and Assessment in Practice: NMC standards for mentors, practice teachers and teachers*. London: NMC.

Nursing and Midwifery Council (NMC) (2008) *Standards to Support Learning and Assessment in Practice: NMC standards for mentors, practice teachers and teachers*, 2nd edn. London: NMC.

Nursing and Midwifery Council (NMC) (2009) *Guidance on Professional Conduct for Nursing and Midwifery Students*. London: NMC.

Quinn, F.M. and Hughes, S.J. (2007) *Quinn's Principles and Practice of Nurse Education*, 5th edn. Cheltenham: Nelson Thornes.

Rogers, C. (1994) *Freedom to Learn*. Englewood Cliffs, NJ: Prentice-Hall.

Wilkes, Z. (2006) The student–mentor relationship: a review of the literature, *Nursing Standard*, 20(37): 42–7.

3 The clinical learning environment

NMC (2008a) domains and outcomes for a mentor related to this chapter

Creating an environment for learning

- Support students to identify both learning needs and experiences that are appropriate to their level of learning

- Use a range of learning experiences, involving patients, clients, carers, and the professional team, to meet defined learning needs

- Identify aspects of the learning environment that could be enhanced – negotiating with others to make appropriate changes

- Act as a resource to facilitate personal and professional development of others

Context of practice

- Contribute to the development of an environment in which effective practice is fostered, implemented, evaluated, and disseminated

(continued)

- Initiate and respond to practice developments to ensure safe and effective care is achieved and an effective learning environment is maintained

Evidence-based practice

- Identify and apply research- and evidence-based practice to their area of practice

- Contribute to strategies to increase or review the evidence base used to support practice

- Support students in applying an evidence base to their practice

Leadership

- Be an advocate for students to support them accessing learning opportunities that meet their individual needs – involving a range of other professionals, patients, clients, and carers

Creating an environment for learning

The fifth domain of the NMC standards for mentors is that of 'Creating a learning environment', which not only entails helping a student identify their learning needs, but also identifying and brokering a range of learning experiences in order for them to meet those needs. This chapter examines that standard and also that of evidence-based practice.

The learning environment is for all

We all, hopefully, contribute to and draw from the learning environment. It is not just a creation for student nurses. We are all students, some of us are on courses, some not – but we are all learners just the same. Colleagues on courses, post-registration students in need of preceptor-ship and mentoring, new healthcare assistants, return-to-practice nurses, nurses from overseas, colleagues from allied professions undertaking insight placements, the list of those benefiting from the learning environment is endless. We must also include ourselves as we strive daily to keep abreast of developments and enhance our knowledge and skills base. So we are all beneficiaries and have a responsibility for creating a culture of debate, enquiry, questioning, reflection, and learning.

Creating a good learning environment is the real substance of mentoring. The student comes to a placement armed with a list of competencies they need to achieve and they will seek to achieve them by experiencing the learning opportunities available under the guidance of their mentor.

While the theory of nursing is taught largely within universities and academic institutions, it is only in the clinical environment that theories can be adequately tested, by putting them into practice. The quality of the placement experience is crucial to this end and central to the quality of that placement experience is the mentor. The rudiments and academic aspects of nursing theory are tested in the fire of reality during clinical experiences, as students discover how the theory needs to be adapted and refined to account for individual variations in circumstance and clinical presentation. It has to be thus, as no two people or situations are completely alike. The placement provides exposure to this variation and the mentor's role is to allow the student to experience its range and so develop the student's skills and confidence in adapting to differing situations.

> *The great advantage of teaching in the clinical area is that it gives access to a key resource which is not available in the classroom, namely direct contact with real patients* (Teesdale 1993, p. 162).

It is also clear that some skills can only be experienced and improved upon in the real world.

> *Students develop their attitudes, competence, interpersonal communication skills, critical thinking and clinical problem solving abilities in the clinical learning environment* (Dunn and Hansford 1997, p. 1299).

Learning to think on your feet under pressure and make decisions in the light of new circumstances can only be done in clinical environments.

Reflecting upon your own training

With a colleague, reflect upon your own training and the clinical learning environments that you experienced. Share the positive and the negative aspects of those clinical areas. Draw up two lists: identify factors that enhanced your learning and made it a good learning environment, and those that detracted from the experience and thus hindered your learning.

Factors that enhance a placement experience

In relation to what makes a good learning environment, research has tended to identify two main factors. The first is linked to the quality of the mentors and staff who are involved, the second to the variety and quality of learning experiences on offer.

Regarding the characteristics of the mentors and staff, student feedback generally identifies what might seem obvious, but is still worth highlighting.

Support

Clinical environments can be strange and stressful places, especially to a novice. A placement might be the new student's first real-life experience of working in a healthcare setting. Many students will be anxious on a new placement and in need of reassurance and encouragement. Even third-year students will feel the need to be supported in the early stages of a placement until they find their feet and become familiar with the routine and staff. This underlines the importance of using associate mentors to widen the range of people the student feels they can access for support. Using healthcare support workers as buddies is another good form of support that also enhances the role and job satisfaction of healthcare support workers (see Chapter 8, 'Helping a student survive a placement'). Similarly, team mentoring fosters the ethos that the student does not just 'belong' to the mentor, but is placed with the team as a whole. The student gains experience of seeing numerous different individual approaches and ways of working, and the assessment process becomes much more objective, as the mentor is able to draw upon a more diverse range of opinion as to the student's ability than if they had tried to 'own' the student. In short, what is required is a whole-team approach whereby all members are happy to have – and keen to help – students. Care must be taken, however, to ensure that students are not 'disowned' by their primary mentor and left to feel as if they have no strong source of support.

Second-year student on surgical ward

I was made to feel welcome and felt like part of the team instantly. I was able to take the opportunity to be involved in many different situations on and off the ward. I got a clearer picture of what happens when a patient is in for surgery and extended my knowledge. I also had the chance to advance on many of my basic nursing skills like washing, dressings, and feeding. I liked the fact I was trusted to choose my own off duty and what shifts I did. The teamwork between the staff members taught me a lot.

First-year student on a medical short-stay ward

As well as basic skills I was able to take part in some other key areas. I was asked to help with things I thought were way beyond me and encouraged to ask questions on rounds. The staff nurses and auxiliaries were nice and friendly and helped me get into the routine quickly and easily. My mentors were very good and although they spent little time actually with me on the placement, they made the effort to ask the other staff to check my performance and abilities to ensure I was able to achieve my outcomes with plenty of evidence.

The possessive student!

Consider the possibility that a student, despite your best efforts, continues to arrange it so that they only work with you and appear to be 'clinging' to you somewhat. How would you approach this situation?

Being friendly, welcoming, and inclusive

Establishing effective working relationships is rightly the first domain of the NMC mentor standards. First impressions count for much and making a student feel welcome and wanted will ease their anxiety. Inclusivity is also important and this should extend to the social milieu of the clinical area. If there is a night out planned, make sure the students are not overlooked. More important than the night out is simply being included in conversations, being included in breaks, and being asked their opinions no matter how 'junior' they are. Again a team approach to mentoring will help foster this sense of belonging. The importance of the way the student is received and welcomed on the first few days cannot be underestimated, as it will make a big impression on and set the tone of the placement for the student. A rapidly assimilated and welcomed student is one who will be able to take advantage of the learning opportunities early on in their placement. Students who feel excluded and unwelcome will likely shy away, withdraw, and have raised anxieties regarding their chances of achieving their objectives.

Third-year student on a medical short-stay ward

I was made to feel like a member of the team rather than just another student (which I haven't experienced anywhere else). The staff were more than happy to show me a range of procedures and explain why and point me towards the relevant literature in support of it.

Third-year student on intermediate care ward

There was an excellent introduction to the placement and all the learning opportunities were explained. All the staff were willing to help me and explain, and my mentor ensured I gained a broad, varied, and interesting experience.

Showing interest and understanding

As above, a little understanding goes a long way. This relates to finding out what stage the student is at in their training and what their own particular needs and interests are. It is important also that the mentor engages with the student early on in order to be able to make a judgement about the student's level of competence, regardless of their stage of training. It's also about acknowledging that students are not just students and that they have other needs and drives. By taking into account childcare or transport issues, as you would with the rest of the ward team, you can help make the student feel respected, acknowledged, and motivated.

Third-year adult acute inpatient nurse

Everyone made me feel part of the team and I practised my clinical skills every day. Any procedure that needed to be carried out they encouraged me to take part. Every day was a new experience.

And another on the same ward on being asked what was good about it . . .

Everything!! This is by far the best placement I have had; everyone works together as a team; the staff are approachable and very supportive. No one minds you asking a million questions and they don't make you feel stupid when you get it wrong!

Giving your time

This is perhaps the hardest thing to achieve. Having set times for teaching or mentoring is usually something of a rarity in most clinical settings and mentors have to be creative. Carving out the time to stop and help the student to reflect upon a learning experience, facilitate a discussion or provide an explanation to a student is often difficult because of the pressures of work. The community mental health nurse, for example, will use the time spent in car journeys to discuss their visits with the student. This is not a luxury afforded to ward-based clinicians. As such, the casual onlooker may get the impression that much nurse education is somewhat chaotic and spontaneous. However, the student experience suggests that simply spending time with their mentor is key to students having a positive experience. It is not so much the need to have lengthy meetings several times a week, although important, but the opportunity for frequent, short interactions, which helps students feel supported. Thus, 'little and often' is usually the order of the day, with perhaps one lengthier meeting each week. With time at such a premium, it is important that mentors fully utilize their colleagues and associate mentors. Not only does this provide the student with more support and teaching, it allows them to experience a broader range of styles and ways of working. The identification of insight visits relevant to the placement will also add structure to experience and make it feel less uncoordinated and chaotic. The following are examples of some innovative methods mentors have tried.

Mentor on acute mental health ward

I feel sorry for some of the students when we are really busy especially on their first days. It can be that we don't get to see much of them so now we plan ahead for this. It doesn't always work, but it has improved things and the student feels less at a loose end. We identify things for them to get involved with and other people to work with in advance every week. So if we are busy they still have things to do. In effect, this spreads the student out over the whole team from the ward clerk to the management. They can learn something from everyone. There is a list of people and services they can contact themselves to arrange visits and insight days. There is also a list of tasks they can undertake when we can't supervise them, such as undertaking a review of the care plans of particular clients to report back on and present.

Surgical ward mentor

If we have two students, they get more support by spreading them across the shifts. Occasionally they are 'shifted' together so that on these shifts they support each other and one mentor keeps an eye on both. If we can foresee quiet periods, we make sure they are both on at that time so that we can get to spend time with them and do their interviews.

Emergency assessment unit nurse

I had to speak to my ward manager and be quite assertive. I had some 'student' time built into the week, usually during lunch periods, and altered my shift pattern slightly so that I had some protected time with my student. It doesn't always come off but it is useful.

District nurse based at multidisciplinary health centre

One way we came up with of giving the students some more time and a bit of structure in what can be a very chaotic centre was to start a prac- tice learning club. Nursing and other students meet with several mentors, other professionals, and the link tutor for an hour and a half a week to discuss cases and different approaches. Sometimes we have speakers in but mainly it is a reflective practice meeting with people discussing their week's practice experience. The students appreciate it by just knowing they will touch base with some support at the same time each week.

Factors that detract from a placement experience

These are largely the opposite of the above, and it isn't rocket science to be able to identify such things as 'feeling unwanted' or a sense of 'being in the way', 'being with staff who don't want to teach', 'not being respected', and 'being made to feel at the bottom of the hierarchy'. Twentyman and

Eaton (2006) suggest that poor treatment of nursing students is common in the workplace for a variety of reasons, including staff shortages, staff sickness, and the fact that some staff can feel threatened by the presence of students. There is much anecdotal evidence, too, that a significant number of students encounter 'mentors' who clearly do not wish to be mentors.

The reluctant mentor!

Thinking about a busy clinical environment, how would you deal with a member of staff who refuses to be a mentor or always avoids it, leaving the burden of responsibility on the shoulders of the other mentors?

There are many other factors that will either add to or detract from a student's placement experience and it is helpful to identify these. Recognising the factors that detract from a placement enables us to eliminate them. The factors listed below will be recognisable to many a student and mentor.

Good and bad learning environments

A following is a selection of responses of nurses reflecting upon their own training a year after they qualified (2007–9):

Good learning environment	Bad learning environment
Consistency	Not enough time with mentor
Resources available	Not expected on placement
Flexibility	Being compared with previous students
Staff approachable	Too many students at the one time
Mentor enthusiasm	Staff shortages
Mentor was patient and understanding	Mentor not interested in students
Student given responsibility	Critical rather than constructive feedback
Identifiable learning opportunities	Used as a pair of hands
Made to feel part of the team	Not welcomed to the team
Sense of humour	Regarded as a healthcare assistant
Encouragement	Clash of personalities
Being respected	Staff unfamiliar with paperwork
Mentor willing to listen	Mentor too busy to give time

(continued)

Given time to reflect	Feeling of not belonging
Teaching sessions on ward	Expectations too high/too low
Shift flexibility	Ward politics/staff disharmony
Insight visits available	Being ignored because it was not my field
Multidisciplinary team working opportunities	No learning opportunities identified
Peer support from other students	
Open-minded staff	

Thankfully, this exercise usually draws out more positives than negatives and on the whole learning experiences are good, but it is sobering that the negatives persist. This highlights the need for good mechanisms for gathering student feedback on placements and acting upon it. The Student Evaluation of Placement proforma towards the end of the chapter outlines a simple but effective way of gathering students' views, and also provides the clinical area with a useful quality monitoring tool.

The impact of things going wrong

First-year student on an adult acute medical ward

I did not feel welcomed when I first met the rest of the team (not very friendly and no introductions apart from two nursing assistants). But I was glad to be put with the nursing assistants for the first few weeks to get used to the basic care and routine. I was told I should be with my mentor but I don't think I saw them more than 20% of the time.

Adult nursing student on first placement

Half the time I didn't have my mentor at all and the first week I didn't even know who it was. I had to go to the ward manager to sort one out for me. I was made to work as a care assistant all the time my mentor was not around. I only actually spent about 3 weeks with her.

Third-year student on a theatre placement

Some staff were very unfriendly. It is difficult going into the theatre environment after being so used to being on the wards, and at times I felt a bit lost and helpless but it would have made me feel better if people introduced themselves and were more welcoming. I always felt it was me having to make the effort. I did my best to fit in.

(continued)

Third-year student on haematology ward

When we got to the placement unit we didn't know where to report for orientation and there were about eight of us for 2 wards, so we were shunted from one place to the other until finally we were told to go back to the School of Nursing.

Learning experiences

A major aspect of a practice placement that plays a large part in students achieving their NMC competencies is the vast number of different learning opportunities there are in any one clinical area. This is true however specialised the area may be. It is a bit of an eye opener to explore the role of the nurse generally and discover the vast array of knowledge and skills that nurses possess. These skills and knowledge bases each represent learning opportunities for mentors to pass on to students.

Role of the nurse

With a few colleagues, take a large sheet of flipchart paper and in the middle draw a small circle and in it write, 'The role of the nurse'.

Create a spider chart by adding a leg for each thing that you think of which is part of the nurse's role, such as medication, care plans, communication skills, breaking bad news, knowledge of the Mental Health Act, pressure care, health promotion, ward management, etc.

This is a sobering exercise when one considers the huge list you are likely to generate. There will be little space left on the page! Figure 3.1 provides an example that could be much expanded.

The example in Figure 3.1 was generated by a group of nurses from several different areas and is by no means exhaustive. Each role listed can be broken down even further into its component parts and its knowledge, skills, and attitude dimensions.

Thinking now about the particular specialty you work in, the following three exercises will help you to explore the range of learning opportunities therein and then break these down even further in order to examine the knowledge, skills, and attitude components of those learning opportunities. The third exercise takes this further still by asking you to map these components against the students' NMC competencies and examine the range of evidence that might be acceptable.

THINGS TO DO

opportunities that can develop in our
clinical area.
- Ward routines.
- Admission / Discharges - critical.
- medicine management.
- Pre and post operative care of pt's.
- Wound care.
- Multidisciplinary team work.
- communication with interprofessional team.

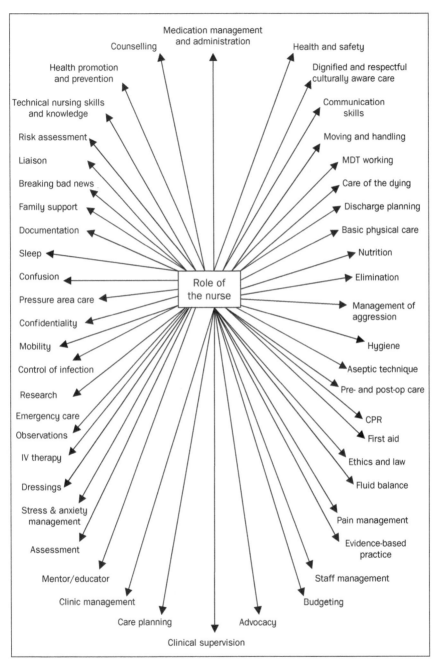

Figure 3.1   Role of the nurse spider chart

The patient's journey

Exercise 3.1

With a group of colleagues, think of a typical patient's journey through your clinical area from admission to discharge.

Using a flipchart, write down every aspect of that patient's care in which the nurse is involved. This will include clinical procedures, assessments, multi-disciplinary working, recording, referral, medication, communication, etc.

Think back to the 'Role of the nurse' exercise and write down everything that you do related to your typical patient.

Again this is usually a bit of an eye opener with respect to the number of procedures, skills, and tasks a nurse must be competent in alongside the breadth of knowledge required to do such. Every aspect of your interventions is also a learning experience for the student nurse. So essentially what you have produced is a list of learning opportunities for students in your clinical area. Figure 3.2 is an example.

The example in Figure 3.2 derives from a group of nurses on a mentor course from similar clinical areas who chose to look at the care of an older person with renal failure and chronic obstructive pulmonary disease. They broke the journey into admission, ward, and discharge phases.

This was a quick 20-minute exercise, but even so it represents a large range of learning opportunities. As a mentor, you could ask your student to undertake a similar exercise.

The second exercise will help you look at the aspects of nursing care in greater detail.

Expanding learning opportunities

Exercise 3.2

Now identify one broad learning experience such as taking a person's blood pressure, giving an injection or encouraging a client with depression to take some nourishment. Again using a flipchart, break this task down into its constituent parts, such as gather equipment together, prepare the trolley, check client's preferences, gain consent, communication skills, etc. You will again be surprised at the number of aspects involved in one simple task, each of which represents a separate learning opportunity. To expand this even further, break the task down into the knowledge, skills, and attitude components that the student nurse will need to perform, display or be aware of.

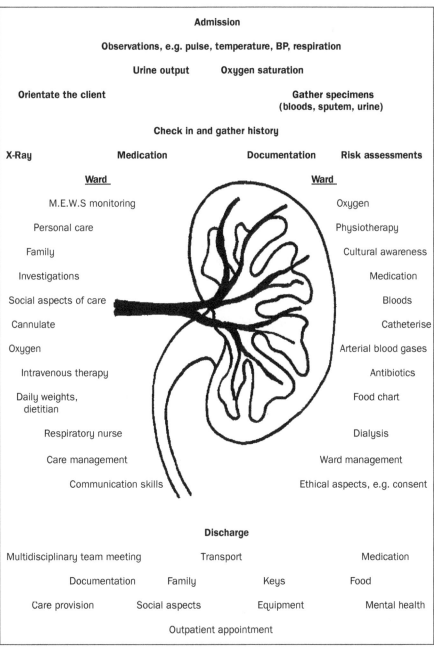

Figure 3.2 Sample patient's journey

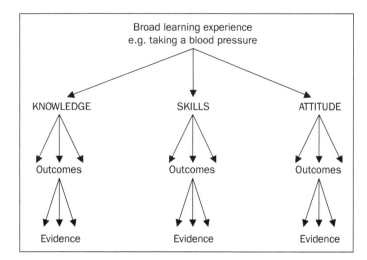

Figure 3.3 Mapping learning experiences

Mapping to outcomes and evidence

Exercise 3.3

Having now generated a long list of aspects of nursing care a student must know and do, map these to the competencies the student has to achieve (see Figure 3.3). The idea here is to see the large range of outcomes a student can achieve in the performance of a single task.

Finally, while doing this exercise, it is worth considering what evidence you would require of the student to be able to assess them as competent.

The exercise in Figure 3.3 can be adapted for use with students as described below.

Exercise for students

Mapping the patient's journey through the clinical area in relation to a given diagnosis is also a useful exercise to give to students, who could then present this on a flipchart to the team. As an exercise in itself, this will allow the student to provide evidence of achieving several of their competencies. Look at one of your student's outcome booklets and try to

(continued)

list these. Such an exercise for the student also allows them to identify gaps in their sphere of knowledge and experience and thus to identify new learning needs. The mentor can then look through this with the student and plan future learning experiences.

Learning resources

The clinical area ideally should have a range of learning resources on hand for students to use to follow up clinical experience. It is important that the student can see the evidence base for the practice they witness and access the latest research used by the specialty.

Alongside the staff group and their special interests, a range of other resources might be considered:

- Ideally there will be a quiet area or room in which resources are located and in which students can work.

- Books and journals are the obvious components and it is useful to get the students themselves to help you build up such a resource. Students can photocopy useful articles they come across and begin to compile a series of files of relevant topics. At least one journal will be of particular relevance to the clinical specialty and if finances are available, a subscription can be taken out. Otherwise, one person can be charged with the task of scanning it each month for relevant articles. If this is not possible, use your university link lecturer to help you identify relevant articles on a regular basis. You could also build up a relationship with the library and your subject specialist to provide you with updates on new books or articles as they are published.

- Health promotion material for patients relevant to the clinical area and clinic/ward information leaflets are useful.

- Also useful is material from national and local organisations or support groups linked to the specialty, alongside government and Department of Health (DH) documents such as policies and National Institute for Health and Clinical Excellence (NICE) guidelines.

- A ward/clinic policy file should be available developed by the local NHS trust.

- Drug companies and equipment manufacturers are always a useful source of information in relation to their products and will often be willing to do short training sessions.

- Cultivate a relationship with your pharmacist and invite them to do an occasional training update on new drugs and refresher sessions on drug administration.

- Student induction packs (see Chapter 2) are also a useful part of the overall resources alongside the placement profiles outlined below.

- Internet access is of course invaluable and there can be a list of credible and useful websites for students to explore.

- Finally, don't forget that the most valuable resource in any clinical area is of course the staff group.

A word of caution!

Occasionally, a student may spend too much time engaged with such resources and divorce themselves from practice. The mentor needs to discuss this with the student and encourage a more appropriate use of their time. Many students have assignments to complete while on placement and are naturally anxious to progress with these, but this should not be at the expense of gaining practice experience. Often the student's withdrawal from clinical work can be a sign of other underlying personal problems and it is important that the mentor acknowledges this and helps the student to access appropriate help if necessary. It is often a sign that the student has not fully integrated into the team and feels ill at ease. The mentor should explore this possibility and put into place remedial measures to ensure the student fully integrates and can thus take full advantage of the practical learning experiences.

Placement profiles

These are written by the clinical staff and are a way of summarising the placement details and giving the student key information about the clinical area and the learning experience they will have and what they can expect. Importantly, they should list the learning opportunities available and include an induction programme for students, a staff profile, and suggested pre-placement reading. The profile should be available as a pack to which the student can refer, and ideally be given to them before the placement begins. Usually this takes the form of a photocopied document or a small file. It needs to be reviewed and updated annually.

Key features of a placement profile include:

- Introduction/welcome statement
- Description of the clinical area and service it provides
- Contact details
- Staff profile and key multidisciplinary team members
- Clinical area philosophy/mission statement
- Induction checklist

- Health and safety, fire, moving and handling issues (in brief)
- Key policies list and location
- Students' responsibilities
- Detailed list of learning opportunities and key skills mapped to competencies
- Link tutor details
- List of insight visits and contact details
- Resources available
- Reading list
- Client/carer information leaflets
- Several key articles
- Copy of last educational audit
- Student complaint statement/procedure
- Student evaluation of placement form

Third-year student on a stroke recovery unit

Specific learning opportunities were identified in the placement information pack alongside what their expectations of a student were. There was background information on strokes and ward routine – this really helped. I also felt supported by the rest of the team when my mentors were not around, and appreciated being able to study their resources now and again to look at the theory and evidence.

Second-year student on same unit

Working with my mentor most of the time ensured continuity and there was an excellent ward arrival pack. I was easily able to achieve all outcomes and had wide and various insight visits.

Insight visits

Insight visits are an integral part of any clinical experience given the multidisciplinary nature of health care today. As a mentor, you could list all the other agencies and professions with whom your clinical area has dealings with, together with their contact details. Students should then be encouraged to arrange any insight visit themselves. Such visits can be used for students to become familiar with these other professionals' roles and their methods of working. The goals and objectives you set for the visits can also be linked to the students' outcomes and competencies. Students can write reflective pieces outlining the learning they have achieved from the visit and use these as evidence within their portfolios.

Links with the School of Nursing/university

It is important to strengthen links with your School of Nursing. Each clinical area should have a named link person from education who has some expertise in your specialty. Their role encompasses supporting both the students and their clinical area and enhancing the learning environment. Ensure that you get to know them and invite them to visit the ward on a regular basis to discuss student-related matters alongside clinical issues. They can help you to build up a resource base and keep you updated clinically. They will also support you in your role as a mentor, especially if there are any difficulties. It is also a good idea to ask the link tutor to help run a journal club for staff and students alike. This meeting can be a regular monthly point of contact and help bridge the theory–practice gap as well as consolidating links with the school. Another good idea is for the link tutor and mentors to hold regular reflective practice sessions for students in the clinical area. The relationship with the school/university should be a two-way process and it is also worth exploring the opportunities for mentors and staff teams to have some input into the taught sessions in the School of Nursing, either giving lectures or running workshops.

Role modelling

There are many opportunities for and instances of informal teaching throughout any shift in every clinical area and indeed this is how most teaching takes place. Students learn by being with and watching their mentors do what they are proficient at. Having a junior student 'shadow' you is an unpressured learning experience for them. Indeed, the previous version of the NMC standards for mentors (NMC 2004) had 'Role modelling' as one of the standards.

This standard was broken down as follows:

- Demonstrate effective relationships with patients and clients

- Contribute to the development of an environment in which effective practice is fostered, implemented, evaluated, and disseminated

- Assess and manage clinical developments to ensure safe and effective care

As a mentor, you will always be a role model. Everything you do is likely to be regarded by students as acceptable practice. Your knowledge, skills, and attitudes will be assimilated. Your professionalism and behaviour in different contexts closely monitored. Taking unacceptable risks or shortcuts, deviating from best practice or policy, and in general acting unprofessionally – all of these things will influence students.

Structured teaching

Alongside the plethora of unstructured informal teaching that occurs naturally, it is good practice to back this up with more formal teaching sessions. Such sessions can be led by nurses or any of the other professionals involved in the clinical area, as well as university staff. The hospital pharmacist, drug company, and equipment representatives are also good sources of training sessions. Many training sessions can be linked to students' outcomes, and you can also develop specific teaching sessions targeting students' competencies. There is often an ongoing round of mandatory training in clinical areas run by the local NHS trust that students may also be able to attend. Sessions such as fire lectures and moving and handling updates can be attended alongside trust staff, which will help the students feel part of the team. Chapter 5 examines teaching in practice in more detail and provides useful guidance on preparing and delivering structured teaching sessions.

Mapping of learning opportunities

For each outcome or competency a student has to achieve, it is possible to generate a list of ways in which the student can achieve it in a specific clinical area. This is a very useful resource for both students and mentors alike. Occasionally, it is not clear what a student can do to achieve an outcome in a particular clinical environment; such a document overcomes this.

Outcome mapping exercise

Choose any student outcome or competency and generate a list of ways in which a student might achieve it in your clinical area. Remember knowledge, skills, and attitudes. You can use this as a base from which to build a complete competency-mapping document for your clinical area.

Here are three examples of competencies mapped for specific clinical areas.

Mental health community experience

Domain 1: Professional values

Competency 1. All nurses must practise with confidence according to *The Code: Standards of conduct, performance and ethics for nurses and midwives* (NMC 2008b).

(continued)

Competency 2.1. Mental health nurses must practise in a way that addresses the potential power imbalances between professionals and people experiencing mental health problems.

Evidence

- Understands the importance of working as part of a multidisciplinary team
- Demonstrates respect for the client and acknowledges their individuality
- Respects the client's rights and choices
- Acknowledges the importance of supervision
- Demonstrates ability to empower the client in decision-making
- Acknowledges own limitations and learning needs
- Observed to ask for guidance when needed

Surgical experience (first year)

Domain 3: Nursing practice and decision-making

Competency 6. All nurses must practise safely by being aware of the correct use, limitations, and hazards of common interventions, including nursing activities.

Evidence

- Considers available resources when planning and carrying out safe patient handling
- Is aware of health and safety policies
- Able to identify and discuss potential hazards in the clinical environment
- Able to describe potential hazards in common procedures
- Can discuss incident reporting procedures
- Reports occurrences that could compromise safety
- Participates in the safe administration of medicines with qualified staff member

Community placement adult year 2

Domain 3: Nursing practice and decision-making

Competency 3.1. Adult nurses must safely use a range of diagnostic skills, employing appropriate technology, to assess the needs of service users.

Evidence

- Demonstrates appropriate communication skills
- Collects data with due regard for client's psychological state
- Performs patient assessment using a range of appropriate tools
- Demonstrates accurate documentation of data
- Gathers information from a range of sources such as family, GP, and other agencies
- Identifies clients' wider community support mechanisms
- Assessments encompass clients' social, psychological, and spiritual needs alongside physical care needs
- Undertakes accurate baseline measurements

It is a daunting task to make a comprehensive list of ways in which students can meet all of their outcomes, but the final document will be extremely useful. Try getting together with mentors from similar areas and the link tutor to form a working group in order to spread the load. Each clinical area in the group can work on different outcomes and the whole can be collated to form a complete outcome-mapping document.

Educational audit

The annual educational audit of the clinical area is a key quality measurement tool for the placement and an ideal opportunity for educators and mentors to reflect upon the effectiveness or otherwise of the placement. The aim is to improve the quality of the placement experience and give recognition to the staff supporting the students. It should highlight good practice, identify areas of concern, and provide an action plan to address any such issues. The audit asks a series of questions regarding the learning experience provided by the clinical area and is undertaken by both educators and clinical staff. The onus is upon the clinical and educational team to provide evidence of how they achieve the standards and criteria set by the audit. The audit should also entail talking with students and mentors in that placement area and also reviewing the student feedback since the last audit. It is also usually the task of the audit to set the numbers of students any one clinical area can accept given the number of mentors they have and the nature of the clinical environment.

Many nursing placement audit tools derive from the guidance set out in *Placements in Focus* (ENB/DH 2001). The key areas examined in audit tools are:

- The safety of the environment
- The learning opportunities
- Student support
- Care is client-centred and respectful

Typical educational audit questions

Safe environment

- How are students made aware of health and safety issues?
- When was the last health and safety inspection?
- What risk assessments are undertaken in the area?
- Are moving and handling policies adhered to and is equipment in place?
- What is the accident/incident procedure where students are involved?
- Are medicines stored as per national guidelines?

Learning opportunities

- What shifts will the students work?
- Is the placement long enough to allow achievement of competencies?
- What learning resources are available?
- What is the philosophy of care?
- Are there sufficient and appropriate learning opportunities?
- Are the staff willing to teach?
- Are students encouraged to contribute to individual care plans?

Student support

- Are students adequately prepared for the placement?
- Is there an orientation/induction pack for students?

(continued)

- Do students have a named mentor and spend sufficient time with them?

- When are students' learning needs identified and achievements assessed?

- Is there opportunity for multidisciplinary working and insight visits?

- Is there evidence of adequate support from the university or School of Nursing?

- Is the number of students allocated appropriate?

- How is student feedback gathered and acted upon?

- Do mentors have access to professional development?

- Is clinical supervision evident?

Respectful and client-centred care

- Does practice respect rights, privacy, dignity, and diversity?

- Do clients consent to the involvement of students?

- Is the care provided client-centred and individualised?

- Are the individual needs of the students themselves taken into account?

It is useful for mentors to examine the educational audit in some detail. The suggestions in the exercise below will facilitate this.

Audit exercises

- Seek out and read the last educational audit for your area.

- Examine the evidence required to meet the questions posed.

- Do you agree with the answers given?

- Have any recommendations been met?

- Ask the School of Nursing for a blank audit tool and audit your own area.

- Ask to sit in on the next audit or one in a different clinical area.

Placements in Focus (ENB/DH 2001) is a guide to auditing clinical areas. It provides an overview of the rationale for practice placements and is a practical guide as to what is expected of placements and what they should provide with respect to learning environments, student support, and assessment of practice in order to ensure quality of provision.

SWOT analysis of the placement area

Undertaking a SWOT analysis as described in Chapter 2 is useful here also. In Chapter 2, the analysis was of your role as a mentor; here it is useful to undertake a SWOT analysis of your clinical environment. Doing so will help you to explore what you have to offer and what gets in your way as you strive to provide the perfect placement experience. Price (2004) offers a very useful model for undertaking this, or you can use the key questions in the education audit for the placement.

SWOT analysis of clinical learning environment: key areas to examine

What are the strengths, weaknesses, opportunities, and threats to your clinical learning environment in relation to the following categories?

- Health and safety of placement
- Learning opportunities
- Care planning
- Evidence-based practice
- Policies/best practice guidelines
- Learning resources
- Student welcome pack and induction programme
- Student support throughout placement/associate mentors
- Multidisciplinary opportunities/insight visits
- Mentor support by management/team
- Mentor having sufficient time for students
- Student feedback is gathered and acted upon

Students' evaluation of placement

Every good placement should be gathering feedback from its students to improve the student experience and enhance their learning opportunities. If this is not being done, then make it your mission to begin gathering such feedback. It also acts as a good quality assurance tool, and is a source of positive feedback to share with others as evidence of good practice. All it needs to be is a sheet of paper with a few pertinent questions as per the proforma below. Simply ask the student to fill it in on their last day.

Student evaluation of placement proforma

To evaluate your placement effectively and help us to improve the learning experience for those who follow, we would value your feedback on the following:

- What preparation for the placement would have been useful?

- In the first week, did you receive an induction and were your learning needs identified with your mentor?

- Did you spend sufficient time with your mentor(s)?

- What were the positive aspects of the placement?

- How do you think this placement could be improved?

- Please add any additional comments you might wish to make.

Physical safety

Physical safety and comfort is an important issue and is a key feature of educational audits of placement areas. *Placements in Focus* (ENB/DH 2001) reminds us that students should not be placed in vulnerable positions and this refers largely to health and safety issues. The placement should be a safe physical environment, having had health and safety inspections annually. This usually incorporates fire safety, storage of dangerous chemicals, and moving and handling practices. However, it is also important to recognise that some clinical areas are prone to violence and that the risks to staff are thus heightened. It is important to ensure that adequate staffing levels and staff training are maintained in such areas and that emergency procedures are in place.

Evidence-based practice

Evidence-based practice is one of the NMC's (2006) competencies for mentors. Its three clauses state that the mentor should be able to:

- Identify and apply research- and evidence-based practice to their area of practice

- Contribute to strategies to increase or review the evidence base used to support practice

- Support students in applying an evidence base to their practice

The clinical environment is where the evidence base is tested and new knowledge generated. New evidence is born of practice and old evidence is updated through practice. At its simplest, evidence-based practice is the use of best evidence to guide and influence current practice and procedures. This is usually achieved by adhering to hospital policy and keeping abreast of new evidence and techniques by reading professional journals and attending courses. Other sources of best practice are national guidelines such as those generated by NICE, Department of Health guidance, conferences, computer databases such as the Cochrane Library or Medline, and not forgetting the feedback from clients and relatives which ought also to be shaping our practice. In this way, the benefits of research are transferred to the clients we treat. The nursing process can be seen as a way in which the raw research evidence is moulded to suit the needs of individual clients and refined in the light of practice experience. Minor changes are made in the application of the evidence and better results are achieved. When this is shared and written up, others try it and so the knowledge develops.

The mentor's role here is to share that expertise and desire for best practice with the student, pointing them towards the sources of best practice and helping them see its practical application and therefore its value.

Best evidence

- What evidence-based practice can you identify in your clinical area?

- What examples of practice in your area require examination of their evidence base?

- What aspects of practice are in need of updating?

- What changes can you make to improve practice? This could be in relation to clinical issues, management and organisation, health promotion/patient information, student teaching, communication, etc.

- Try to identify possible areas for nursing research within your clinical area.

- Is there something you are doing that is worth writing up and sharing with others?

The proficient nurse ensures they are using evidence-based practice but the expert nurse generates new evidence. The excitement of being in an environment where new knowledge is being generated can only be inspirational for student nurses. Such nurses are those who contribute to and write articles, attend journal clubs, attend and present at conferences, and derive satisfaction from pushing the boundaries of their expertise further.

The long history of health research has slowly grown to incorporate nurse researchers, but most clinicians still do not become active researchers, anecdotally through lack of time and management support. What appears at first to be a daunting process can however be achieved by using a simple action research framework. The action research method closely resembles the nursing process in that both are similar cycles of observing, planning, acting, and evaluating. Indeed, one could argue that nursing is a form of action research in practice.

Action research

Developed originally from the work of Kurt Lewin (1946), a social psychologist working in the 1940s, action research is essentially a method of research that aims to change practice rather than merely generate new knowledge. Its other significant difference from mainstream research is that the researchers work in the situation being researched; in effect, they research themselves in action. In this way, the research is undertaken and owned by practitioners whose sole aim is to improve their own practice.

In many ways, it closely mirrors the nursing process because it encompasses a cycle of activity that becomes a spiral of ongoing evaluation and improvement. It is also essentially reflective in nature.

Figure 3.4 mirrors the problem, plan, action, and evaluate nursing process cycle. The idea is that by reflecting upon that which we want to improve, we gain new understanding and have new ideas or theories, often just minor changes that we put into action and then evaluate, and so on. If it brings about an improvement or gives new insights into current practice, it should be shared via publication so that others might try it. So the cycle can be seen simply as Figure 3.5.

The key stages in the action research process are:

1. Reflect upon what you want to improve

2. Record and describe what is happening now

3. Do a literature search to see what others have done

4. Plan a change

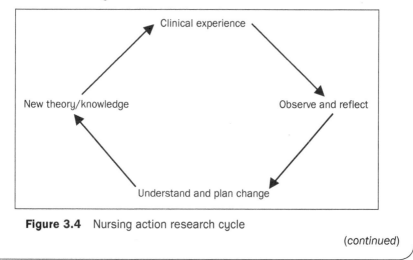

Figure 3.4   Nursing action research cycle

(continued)

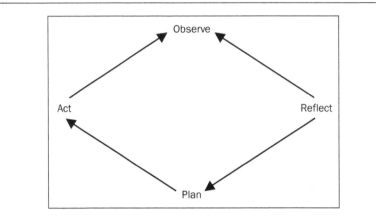

Figure 3.5 Simplified nursing action research cycle

5. Implement it

6. Observe

7. Evaluate its results

8. Amend the plan

9. Repeat the cycle

It is a simple process but an effective one that can help nurses to improve practice and share those improvements via publication. Mentors undertaking action research based upon their practice will be a source of inspiration to student nurses, instilling in them a sense of what is possible given enthusiasm and commitment.

First-year adult field student on older adult mental health ward

There is an excellent structure in place to support and facilitate the student's learning. All student material provided was relevant, recent, and evidence based. Documentation is provided on the first day. The mentor and their associate seem to be assigned well in advance of the student's arrival in the area.

Mentor's evaluation of placement

Student nurses undertake an evaluation of their placement experience after each placement. This information is used as a quality measure and also as a vital feedback mechanism for the placement to see how they are doing and how they might improve their learning environment and experience.

Of equal value would be a mentor evaluation of the placement and their mentoring experience.

Such evaluations are rarely undertaken, but it would be a useful quality assurance measure for mentors and their associates to hold brief post-placement post mortems as to how well a placement went. These can examine the student feedback and the mentors' own views to determine what adjustments may be needed to the learning environment, learning experiences, organisation, student support, resources, and so on. It would be useful for the link tutor to be involved too, so that issues related to students can be addressed in a timely fashion. Such meetings held at the end of the placement need only be brief but will allow for any suggestions to be implemented before the arrival of the next student.

Such an evaluation could also detail difficulties encountered in performing the role of mentor, what went well, what got in the way, what could be improved, and so on. This would be a good managerial tool for appraising the practicalities of mentoring and identifying the support mentors need. It might also be useful in highlighting for the university aspects such as the students' preparedness or otherwise for the placement and identifying any knowledge gaps that need attention prior to a student being placed on that particular placement.

Exercise

Draw up a list of questions for an evaluation of placement by mentors.

Conclusion: putting it all together

By bringing together all the ideas discussed in this chapter, it is possible to identify a list of positive factors in a learning environment.

Checklist of qualities in a good clinical learning environment

- A written philosophy of care
- National and local policies and procedures available and adhered to
- A team leader who is enthusiastic about students
- A welcoming, democratic team which encourages questions
- Good team spirit/relationships/communication
- A safe environment
- Students are encouraged to make pre-placement visits
- Associate mentoring/team mentoring
- Healthcare assistant buddies

- Close clinical supervision
- Learning resources and study area are available
- Structured teaching sessions
- Staff can access professional development/training
- Practice is evidence based and best practice guidelines are available
- Practice respects rights, dignity, privacy, and diversity
- There is a welcome/induction/orientation pack/placement profile
- Learning opportunities are identified and mapped to competencies
- Learning needs are identified and regularly reviewed
- A range of insight visits are identified
- Staff value learning and time is allowed for reflection
- Feedback is frequent and assessment ongoing
- The area is regularly audited for education
- Mentors are regularly updated
- Mentors are allocated prior to placement
- Multidisciplinary working opportunities are evident
- Student feedback is collected and acted upon
- Client satisfaction data are gathered
- Good (named) links are held with the university/School of Nursing

Summary

This chapter has:

- Highlighted the factors that enhance a learning environment
- Identified what can detract from it
- Examined the breadth of learning opportunities and mapping them to the students' competencies
- Discussed the importance of evidence-based practice and the usefulness of action research
- Highlighted the importance of placement evaluation

Having discussed the qualities of the clinical learning environment, it is now logical to explore the teaching that goes on in that environment in more detail. The next chapter examines the theory that underpins that teaching and learning.

Further reading

Gopee, N. (2008) *Mentoring and Supervision in Healthcare*. London: Sage. See Chapter 4: 'The clinical setting as an effective learning environment'.

Hinchliff, S. (ed.) (1999) *The Practitioner as Teacher*, 3rd edn. London: Baillière Tindall. See Chapter 1: 'Creating a learning environment'.

Jackson, D. and Mannix, J. (2001) Clinical nurses as teachers: insights from students of nursing in their first semester of study, *Journal of Clinical Nursing*, 10(2): 270–77.

Morton-Cooper, A. (2000) *Action Research in Health Care*. Oxford: Blackwell. Chapter 1 is a useful introduction to the history of action research, and its basic principles.

Murray, C., Rosen, L. and Staniland, K. (2010). *The Nurse Mentor and Reviewer Update Book*. Maidenhead: Open University Press.

Oliver, R. and Endersby, C. (1994) *Teaching and Assessing Nurses: A handbook for preceptors*. London: Baillière Tindall. See Chapter 8: 'The clinical learning environment'.

Papp, I., Markkanen, M. and von Bonsdorff, M. (2003) Clinical environment as a learning environment: student nurses' perceptions concerning clinical learning experiences, *Nurse Education Today*, 23(4): 262–8.

Twentyman, M. and Eaton, E. (2006) Enhancing support for student nurses in the clinical setting, *Nursing Times*, 102(14): 35. This is an excellent summary of various factors that help students achieve positive placement experiences.

West, S., Clark, T. and Jasper, M. (2007) *Enabling Learning in Nursing and Midwifery Practice: A guide for mentors*. Chichester: Wiley. See Chapter 3: 'The reflective mentor: the student's perspective of their needs in the practice setting'.

References

Dunn, S.V. and Hansford, B. (1997) Undergraduate nursing students' perceptions of their clinical learning environment, *Journal of Advanced Nursing*, 25(6): 1299–306.

ENB/Department of Health (ENB/DH) (2001) Principles and guidance for good practice, Chapter 3 in *Placements in Focus: Guidance for education in practice for health care professions*. London: English National Board for Nursing, Midwifery and Health Visiting/Department of Health.

Lewin, K. (1946) Action research and minority problems, *Journal of Social Issues*, 2(4): 34–46.

Nursing and Midwifery Council (NMC) (2004) *Standards for the Preparation of Teachers of Nurses, Midwives and Specialist Community Public Health Nurses*. London: NMC.

Nursing and Midwifery Council (NMC) (2006) *Standards to Support Learning and Assessment in Practice: NMC standards for mentors, practice teachers and teachers*. London: NMC.

Nursing and Midwifery Council (NMC) (2008a) *Standards to Support Learning and Assessment in Practice: NMC standards for mentors, practice teachers and teachers*, 2nd edn. London: NMC.

Nursing and Midwifery Council (NMC) (2008b) *The Code: Standards of conduct, performance and ethics for nurses and midwives*. London: NMC.

Price, B. (2004) Evaluating your learning environment, *Nursing Standard*, 19(5).

Teesdale, K. (1993) Optimum use of limited resources: structured teaching in the clinical area, *Professional Nurse*, December: 162–8.

Twentyman, M. and Eaton, E. (2006) Enhancing support for student nurses in the clinical setting, *Nursing Times*, 102(14): 35.

4 Teaching and learning theory

Key points

- We each have our own personal learning style

- Understanding how people learn helps us to adjust our teaching appropriately

- Teaching and learning theories can inform our teaching but they must be adapted to the subject and the needs of the learner

- Bloom's (1956) taxonomy is especially useful for teaching nursing

NMC (2008) domains and outcomes for a mentor related to this chapter

Facilitation of learning

- Use knowledge of the student's stage of learning to select appropriate learning opportunities to meet their individual needs

- Facilitate selection of appropriate learning strategies to integrate learning from practice and academic experiences

- Support students in critically reflecting upon their learning experiences in order to enhance future learning

Apart from facilitating learning experiences, key elements of these competencies mean that we must assess what the student already knows (the stage they are at), understand how they learn, and help them to reflect upon their learning experiences.

Theory and practice

How does theory help?

An understanding of the variety of ways in which people learn should enable the teacher to adapt their methods to suit each individual student, thereby maximizing the learning that occurs.

No rules, just guidelines!

Teaching should almost be second nature to nurses, as the teaching process all but mirrors the nursing process. A learner's needs are assessed, a teaching plan is then formed, implemented, and finally evaluated through assessment of the learner. Teaching and learning theories are useful in showing us how different approaches can inform and improve the way we teach in different situations and with different subject matter and different learners. The teacher should not adhere strictly to any one approach, but rather be eclectic and use the best principles of each. Each theory naturally lends itself to certain subject matter.

The same approach should be adopted in relation to learning styles; they are there to inform and help us to adapt our teaching techniques to the individual needs of the learner. As learners, we may have one preferred way of learning but will often swing from one learning style to another depending upon what we are trying to learn at the time. The practice reality for teaching is similar to nursing: you adapt to the needs of individuals. Having said that, teaching is also about taking people out of their comfort zone and showing them new ways of learning, as opposed to finding out how the learner prefers to learn and sticking with it. In this way, teachers can help learners to develop a more 'rounded' approach to learning so that they are helped to develop their learning skills by using methods and techniques they are less comfortable with. There are many factors that affect teaching and learning, and as such the theory provides us with no rules for teaching, just good guidelines.

Factors affecting learning

Thinking about your own previous learning experiences, list the factors that affected your learning in relation to the following:

1. The environment

2. The learner

3. The teacher

4. The methods

Teaching and learning theories

There are many different theories and models of learning, but the three major theories are behaviourist, humanistic, and cognitive. No one theory holds the truth, but each is useful in different ways and in different settings. The teacher, then, needs to be eclectic and choose a mixture of approaches to suit the needs of individual students and the material being taught.

Behaviourist theories

Behaviourist teaching is based upon the key concepts of stimulus, response, and conditioning. Two of the key behaviourist principles are those of 'classical conditioning' and 'operant conditioning'. The work of early behaviourists such as J.B. Watson showed that the more a stimulus and response occurred, the more it became part of our behaviour pattern. We can, however, be conditioned to respond to stimuli. It could be said that the teacher attempts to condition the student to respond or act in a certain way. In his classic experiments, Skinner (1938) trained pigeons to operate a lever to obtain food. The food acted as the reinforcer for the pigeon's behaviour. In teaching, it is often the teacher's praise that is the positive reinforcement, alongside the student's sense of satisfaction or pleasure at succeeding. It's a simple basic principle but a strong one – the more you reward a behaviour, the more it will be done. Repetition is also a key feature of behaviourist theory, as Watson showed, and behaviourist approaches to teaching are very good for teaching manual and skills-based tasks, where mere repetition can lead to mastery. A good example here is the giving of an intramuscular injection. This is a task that induces apprehension in many student nurses. The rudiments of the technique are quite simple but it is only by practising that mastery can be gained. Lectures here will do little good after the principles of the technique are learnt; what is needed is plenty of practice in the skills laboratory. Here, under guidance, the student can become familiar with handling the syringe and needle and repeat the actions of the process of injecting as many times as they want. This repetition and your praise will enable the student to move towards competence.

Much like Skinner, in behaviourist teaching the teacher is in control, directing the learning, and the student is largely the passive receiver. The two behaviourist principles of classical and operant conditioning are examined below.

Classical conditioning

Classical conditioning derives from the work of Pavlov and his dog experiments. He believed that behaviour was a reaction to stimuli. We are born with certain innate, unconditioned responses, such as salivating at the sight of food. Pavlov believed that all other behaviour was conditioned or learnt. Food is an unconditioned stimulus (US). Dogs naturally (unconditionally) salivate at the sight of food and this is an unconditional response (UR). Pavlov found that if he then rang a bell every time he fed them, he could eventually make the dogs salivate just by ringing the bell in the absence of any food. The bell becomes a conditioned stimulus (CS) and the salivation is now a conditioned response (CR). This is an example of classical conditioning or, put another way, learning by association.

(continued)

Operant conditioning

This term refers to the fact that Skinner was interested in behaviours that 'operated' on the environment. He believed that it was the outcomes of behaviour that determined whether or not it was repeated. Skinner's pigeons were conditioned to push a lever to obtain food. The food was the reward that reinforced the behaviour. Operant conditioning, then, is when behaviour is modified by its consequences, i.e. reinforced by reward or weakened by punishment. Skinner also demonstrated that rewards were better at shaping behaviour than negative responses such as punishments.

Social learning theory

Bandura (1977) suggests that learning can take place simply by being with others and watching them – in short, people learn from one another via observation and modelling. You are also more likely to copy and adopt the behaviour and attitudes of those you respect and admire. This can be seen as a variant of behaviourist approaches. The student observes the competent nurse, whom they hold in high regard, they see the outcomes of that nurse's behaviour as positive and try to copy their behaviour, skills, and attitudes. If that nurse then gives them positive reinforcement through praise, the skills and attitudes are likely to be consolidated and reinforced even more. Thus the nurse is in a powerful position here as a role model. However, students can also learn undesirable behaviours and attitudes in this way.

Key principles of behaviourist theory

- New behaviours can be learned.
- Repetition is important in learning, especially for skills.
- Practice in varied contexts reinforces learning and widens its application.
- Positive reinforcement and praise cement learning and shape behaviour.
- It is important to give feedback (reinforce) as close to the event as possible.
- Do not reinforce undesirable behaviours.
- Active learning is better than passive learning.

Humanistic theories

Humanistic theories take into account underpinning feelings, attitudes, and values when examining knowledge and skills and suggest that the rationale for learning is personal growth. These theories see the teacher as a facilitator rather than a pedagogue and also view experiential learning as especially useful. Humanistic approaches are particularly useful in teaching ethics and attitudes in nursing. One of the key features of the approach is the importance of creating a democratic, student-centred, welcoming, and safe teaching environment. Students will, for example, engage much more in a discussion taking place in a respectful, democratic environment than one in which humanistic principles are not apparent.

Carl Rogers

In relation to his theories on counselling, Rogers believed in a safe atmosphere in which people felt able to express themselves openly. Rogers argues that the same ethos is important for education. Such an uncritical atmosphere fosters confidence and boosts self-esteem in the learner, as they feel free to explore new knowledge without fear of reproach. It is often said that a good learning environment is one in which you are not afraid to ask questions for fear of being criticised. A learning environment where a learner feels able to speak their mind and air their views is a healthy one. Thus the teacher provides a safe, encouraging environment, guides the student to resources and opportunities, and facilitates the student's exploration of them. Rogers also argues that the more interest a teacher shows in a student and the more positive feedback they are given, the greater will be the student's self-confidence and self-esteem and thus their desire and ability to learn. This is also a form of behaviourism (the interest of the teacher is a reward) and its power is seen if we consider the opposite: if you criticise someone often enough, you will put them off completely. By constantly finding fault in a student, the mentor will demoralise the student and make them withdraw from learning opportunities.

Abraham Maslow

Maslow's (1987) 'hierarchy of needs' helps us to understand the role motivation plays in learning (Figure 4.1). According to Maslow, basic needs have to be met before higher-order needs such as learning. Put simply, you cannot enjoy listening to your favourite piece of music if you are very hungry.

Learning is a higher-order need, but a lower priority in the immediate survival stakes, so we need to take care of the lower-order needs first before the learner can concentrate on learning. Similarly if a learner feels uneasy or anxious in a group, or does not feel an equal member of the group, their learning will be compromised because their security and belonging needs will not be met.

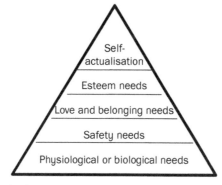

Figure 4.1   Maslow's hierarchy of needs

Maslow's hierarchy of needs in relation to education

Physical needs:	The room is warm, the learner is fed and not tired.
Safety needs:	It is a secure area where the student doesn't feel threatened.
Belonging needs:	The student feels welcome and wanted. They feel they are of equal status and belong to the group.
Esteem needs:	The student feels encouraged and their confidence is boosted by praise and positive reinforcement. Their contribution is valued.
Self-actualisation:	The student learns and moves towards maximising their potential and achieving their goals and ambitions.

Maslow's hierarchy is not always borne out, as in the case of many artists and writers who lived in abject poverty with their basic needs often unmet but who nevertheless were extremely creative. However, as a general principle it remains valuable. Our patients, for example, will not be able to take on board our health education while they are in acute pain or highly anxious. The student nurse will not be able to fully concentrate on the procedure if they have not eaten or slept very well for a while, or feel anxious about the new placement because they haven't settled in.

Adult learning (andragogy)

The concept of adult learning also falls under humanistic approaches.

Andragogy means 'relating to adult learning' and is largely derived from the work of the humanistic educator Malcolm Knowles (1990). Knowles suggests that there are four basic differences between adult learners and child learners and these form the four key principles of andragogy:

Self-concept

Adults take responsibility for their own learning. We become less dependent and more self-directed in our learning as we mature and less reliant upon the teacher, thus learning becomes more student-centred. As adults, we need to be more involved in the planning and evaluation of our learning.

Experience

As adults, we have a range of past experiences and prior knowledge and use this as a resource for learning and to direct our future learning.

Readiness to learn

Adult learners are more likely to be in education voluntarily. As adults, we are more willing to take responsibility for our own learning and tend to focus more on that which has direct relevance to our lives. Open discussion is more achievable.

Orientation to learning

Adults try and apply their learning to life and tend to become more problem-focused rather than content-oriented.

Knowles' principles and assertions of differences between adult and child learners have been the subject of some debate and criticism: there will always be some adults who are unmotivated for example, but one must see Knowles' principles as generalisations rather than rules. In doing so, they can help inform the way in which we relate to and teach our student nurses, most of whom we will readily regard as adult learners.

Pedagogy

Pedagogy can be seen as the opposite of andragogy and it is generally regarded as relating to teaching children in schools. It is descriptive of the traditional approach to teaching, which regards the teacher as the font of all knowledge and upon whom the student is dependent. The teacher decides what will be learned as well as where, when, and how it will be learned. In general, the student's prior knowledge is not taken into account or acknowledged and by and large the student is driven by pressure from the teacher or assessments. One can see that in modern schooling beyond the infant years, teaching methods have moved on from this somewhat crude view of teaching and embraced many aspects of the andragogical approach, by regarding children as more autonomous and mature and having valid life experiences.

Key principles of humanistic theory

- Each learner is seen as an individual.
- Learning is self-directed.
- The teacher is a resource and facilitator of opportunities.
- Anxiety affects learning.
- Learners' self-esteem is important.
- The atmosphere and climate of the classroom are important.
- The relationship with the teacher is important.
- People learn best by participation and cooperation.

Cognitive theories

Cognitive theories of learning hinge on the belief that learning involves mental processes, such as perception, reasoning, memory, and information processing. The principles of cognitive approaches are especially useful in teaching theory, via the use of problem-solving approaches, analysis, and experimentation.

Bruner

Bruner's (1966) contribution to the debate might seem obvious but it highlights key principles that shouldn't be ignored. Bruner's theory of instruction consists of four elements:

1. He believed that learners have to be ready to learn and that teaching should be focused on problem-solving, which will stimulate the learner's curiosity. It is far more interesting to have to use theory than merely learn it; in this way, a case scenario will bring the theory to life.

2. The teaching should be structured and presented in a way that makes it easy to understand. It should incorporate demonstrations, images, and diagrams. An unstructured lecture, for example, which merely presents a mass of information verbally, is unlikely to be remembered as well as one that is presented using a variety of methods such as pictures, demonstrations, and case scenarios.

3. The teaching should be logically sequenced so as to form a progression, allowing the learner to build upon what they already know. For example, explaining the steps of giving an intramuscular injection in

sequence, as opposed to randomly examining the various aspects and considerations.

4. The motivation of the learner is important and comes initially from the teacher's praise (extrinsic) and later the student's own satisfaction (intrinsic) at solving a problem. Mentors may have to motivate some students initially if, for example, they are in a non-field placement and not particularly interested in that area of nursing. Having pointed out the relevance and learning opportunities related to all nursing fields, most students will begin to motivate themselves as they start to see the relevance.

Ausubel

Ausubel's (1978) assimilation theory (a logical progression on Bruner) rests on the assertion that new knowledge always builds upon existing knowledge. New information is incorporated into the learner's already existing cognitive structure. This underlines the importance of a logical progression in learning. New knowledge is more easily assimilated if it already has a familiar concept upon which it fits or builds. Thus the skills are first taught in the lab and then tested out in real life on placement. Bits of new knowledge or variations in the skill are easily added to what is already known. Learning a new variation of a technique is easier than learning a technique from scratch. Another good example is giving a student reading to undertake prior to a lecture or skill session. The lecture will make more sense as the student will already have a base upon which to build. Having that little bit of prior knowledge aids retention of the material to be taught. Such preparation prior to teaching is referred to as an 'advance organiser'. Advance organisers can also help to consolidate and revise learnt material, via engaging with the material in different ways (e.g. bullet point summaries, diagrams, mind and concept maps, timelines). These are good learning tools to use with students on placement by asking them to create, for example, a timeline of a patient's illness and treatment for life, or a mind map of the issues relating to consent.

> *The most important single factor influencing learning is what the learner already knows* (Ausubel 1968: vi).

Gestalt

Gestalt psychologists believe that if you break things down too far, it becomes hard to see the full picture. They believe that 'the whole is greater than the sum of its parts'. Gestalt suggests then that learners learn best when they can see the 'big picture' and where the learning fits into it. Gestalt learning theory is also learning by insight. You gain insight by putting the disparate elements of a problem together and finally it clicks and you can see the big picture, what Gestalt psychologists call the 'aha' moment. The insight then is fostered typically by problem-solving exercises, group discussions, and projects. Case scenarios and discussions of critical incidents are useful, leaving the students to try and resolve the situation under scrutiny. Often, students cannot see the wood for the trees and can struggle with blind theory but when they are asked to engage with that theory in relation to a case scenario and are invited to work on it, bells begin to ring (the 'aha' moment) and connections begin to be made as the theory slowly reveals the sense it makes.

There is an obvious dichotomy here between 'serialist' (e.g. Ausubel) and 'wholist' (e.g. Gestalt) approaches to learning. Some learners will prefer to see the bigger picture while others will prefer to build their knowledge step by step. There will also be certain subject matter that is more easily assimilated through a wholist approach, such as humanities, and other subject matter that is more easily assimilated via a step-wise progression, such as information technology skills. The skilled teacher will seek to incorporate a blend of both approaches in their practice.

Experiential learning and reflection

Experiential learning is learning by doing and then reflecting upon it to explore it and gain new insights. This is a key feature of the action research cycle as described in Chapter 3 and Kolb's (1984) learning cycle (see below). Critical incident analysis is another example of this, where a concrete experience is examined via a reflective cycle in order to generate new insights. The Gibbs (1988) model of reflection is a useful example of a reflective tool that can be used by mentors to get students to examine clinical experiences. Reflection is a key feature of portfolio work and of nurse education generally. There is a more detailed discussion highlighting the importance of reflection in Chapter 7.

Dewey

Dewey (1974) was a wide-ranging intellectual thinker who suggested that the only way to test theory and philosophy was by its practical results. Because of this, he became known as a pragmatist. His influence upon education was in stressing the importance of the teacher. He also believed that education should be active and that learning should involve real-life tasks and ultimately have an impact upon life and communities. As such, he was at the forefront of experiential education and schemes such as outward bound.

Key principles of cognitive theory

- Material should be presented in a logical sequence.

- The learner's participation is important.

- Learning moves from the simple to the complex, building upon the previous step.

- New learning is linked to existing knowledge.

- Goal-setting by the learner is an important motivator.

- The learner needs to see the bigger picture.

- Teachers should demonstrate the links between the whole and its parts.

- Reflection leads to insight.

Student reflections

These reflections from students show that while theory is important, it relies upon the mentor to apply it and create a good learning experience.

Third-year student on a medical ward

I was encouraged to ask questions by the whole team and allowed to participate in new situations. I was supported and encouraged by all staff to reach my potential without feeling pressured. They let me go at my own pace and allowed me time to settle into the ward.

Third-year student on a medical ward

The nurses were always willing to work with students and give us the opportunities which arose. Even though it was hectic and busy there was always someone around if you needed them. They let you get on with it and this helped you to build up your confidence. I was never afraid to ask if I wasn't sure of something.

Second-year student on a cancer ward

I was made to feel welcome by the members of the team and even though I had transport issues they made it so I could fit in and feel part of it. They helped me to feel at ease when developing my nursing skills even though I went wrong sometimes.

(continued)

Third-year student on a medical ward

> I knew most of the basic skills and wanted to start learning more but felt I lacked confidence. The mentor was very supportive and understood where I was at. She showed me a few simple tasks that I was responsible for and this built my confidence. This gave me something to do and avoided the feeling of being lost – it made me feel useful. She then explained the evidence base to me. Having gotten more confident I observed her do a dressing, doing it myself the next day with her supervising. She told me to get the trolley ready, making me think in advance what I had to do when I was with the patient. If I got anything wrong, she calmly explained it. She used simple steps but over the placement I did more and more.

Third-year student on forensic mental health placement

> Both my mentors were good. The first, because she took the time to get to know me and my strengths and weaknesses, so she knew how best to teach me. She gave me a good role model: conscientious, cool-headed, and well read. The second pushed me to do what I was afraid to do and put me in contact with others who could help me to make the most of the placement.

Learning styles

As with learning theories there are a range of ideas relating to learning styles, each of which can inform our teaching methods. Educationalists believe that we all have our own particular learning style, a way of taking on board information that is unique to us. Some of us prefer to learn by listening and taking notes and reading around the subject as much as we can; others prefer a more hands-on approach to learning and like to watch demonstrations and practise themselves. Some of us respond better to a very visual style of teaching, whereas others prefer to listen. Some of us like to join in and participate, while others like to quietly soak it up.

The key protagonists with respect to learning styles are David Kolb, and Peter Honey and Alan Mumford (1988) whose work developed from that of Kolb. Kolb developed a theory of a learning cycle and identified different types of learning preferences. Honey and Mumford went on to develop their own version of these 'learning styles' and identified four key styles. Another learning style theory is the visual, auditory, kinaesthetic learning style, or VAK. Criticisms have been levelled at these theories, as you will find later in the chapter, but the crucial point for mentors is the practical one that for students to learn best we must first identify how they prefer to learn.

The work of Kolb

Kolb (1984) was essentially interested in how we learn from the concrete experiences we have. He argues that the way we perceive and process information determines how we learn and therefore the learning style we adopt. Thus we develop preferences for different ways of learning (i.e. learning styles) in much the same way that we have different communication or leadership styles and dispositions to behave in certain ways. The practical application of this idea is that if teaching is consistent with the learner's learning style, the potential for learning is increased.

Kolb identifies a cycle of learning that consists of four key stages, as shown in Figure 4.2. Individuals immerse themselves in an experience, for example they perform a task and then they observe and reflect upon its effect. Next they form thoughts and concepts about the task and its effectiveness and so they begin to understand it better. They then apply the refined knowledge in new situations and actively experiment with it and use it for problem-solving. In this way, it can be seen as a cycle of learning that is ongoing and continuously refined – in effect, it is a spiral of learning, hopefully increasing our knowledge with each cycle. There is a direct parallel here with Lewin's action research cycle (Lewin, 1946) (see Chapter 3). You will also note the close similarity with the nursing process (see Figures 4.3 and 4.4). Kolb suggests that by going through the cycle several times, we gain sufficient understanding of it to imbue us with the ability to anticipate the effects of the action in different circumstances.

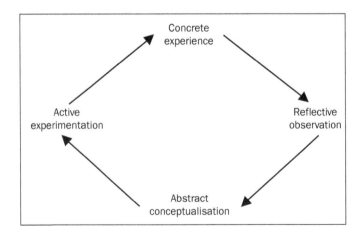

Figure 4.2 Kolb's learning cycle

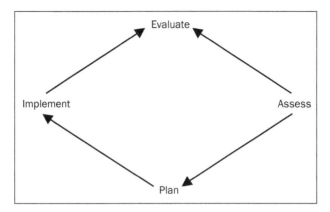

Figure 4.3 The nursing process

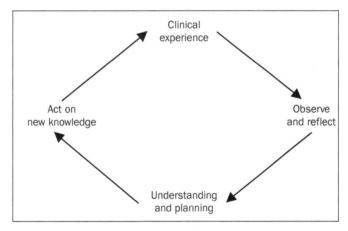

Figure 4.4 The nursing process and Kolb's learning cycle combined

This is somewhat akin to the intuition of experienced nurses as described by Benner (1984).

Kolb sees the stages of his cycle as abilities and suggests that people learn best by going through all four stages – that is, concrete experience, reflective observation, abstract conceptualisation, and active experimentation. He also says that most people develop a preference for using one or two of these stages or abilities, as opposed to being gifted in all. Kolb suggests that one can identify four basic types of learning style, each favouring a blend of two of the stages or abilities.

Kolb produced a questionnaire or learning style inventory that can be used to ascertain which learning style an individual shows a preference for. He also describes the characteristics of these four learning styles (see below). Others have subsequently amended his theory, each adding their own interpretation.

Divergers (concrete experience/reflective observation)

Divergers like to use their imagination, observe and try to see things from different angles. They like to gather much information and generate ideas. They are said to have broad cultural interests.

Assimilators (abstract conceptualisation/reflective observation)

Assimilators have a liking for theory and logic and thinking things through. They are said to have the ability to create theoretical models.

Convergers (abstract conceptualisation/active experimentation)

Convergers like problem-solving and practical application of concepts. They are said to prefer working with objects rather than people and do well on conventional tests.

Accommodators (concrete experience/active experimentation)

Accommodators are doers and risk-takers with a preference for hands-on experiences and practical sessions. They are said to be good at adapting to new situations and putting ideas into action and are supposed to be intuitive.

Kolb's influences

The work of Kolb has helped foster today's interest in experiential learning, but his influences were Dewey (1933) and Lewin (1946), both of whom were early pioneers in this field.

Honey and Mumford

These two educational psychologists developed a model of learning styles largely based on the work of Kolb. They adapted Kolb's four learning styles and called them Activists, Reflectors, Pragmatists, and Theorists. They also suggest that by and large we are unaware of our preferred learning style and can, in fact, have more than one. Much like Kolb, you can complete a questionnaire to check what your preferred learning style is (see Further reading).

Honey and Mumford (1988) and their interpreters attribute certain characteristics to each of the learning styles.

Activists

Activists learn best by being actively involved; they like to immerse themselves in new experiences and enjoy being thrown in at the deep end. They learn by doing rather than reading or listening and are said to be open-minded and receptive to simulations, case studies, and role modelling. They are also open to new experiences and enjoy a degree of risk or challenge. They like to be at the centre – chairing meetings and leading. However, they can suffer from insufficient planning and be too hasty and are said to often neglect subjects that don't interest them. When teaching an activist, you need to make sure they are involved, so give them case studies to work on and problems to solve or projects to report back on.

Theorists

Theorists like to consider problems, they strive to understand concepts and integrate them into their thinking. They learn through logic and facts, via lectures and reading, seeking to understand the theory behind and reason for what they observe. They are said to prefer to do things in a logical order and in set ways, being somewhat rigid and cautious. They will need much information before they are convinced to act. When teaching a theorist, you will need to supply them with a good reading list and get them to follow things up. It is useful to ask them to write up their findings and prepare a summary or synopsis to report back to others.

Reflectors

Reflectors learn best by standing back and observing and reflecting upon what they see and experience. Reflective writing and journals are likely to help them learn. Said to be cautious, they learn best by watching and thinking and talking things through rather than participating. They like to consider all angles and review the evidence before coming to any conclusion. Creative and easy-going, they will listen to others but can be worried by time pressures. When teaching a reflector, you will need to facilitate discussion groups and set tasks that require a reflective account to be produced and shared.

Pragmatists

Pragmatists like to try out new ideas and engage in problem-solving. They learn by applying things to practice, testing and experimenting to see if they work. They are receptive to role modelling. They like to 'get things done'. Practical and well organised, they set goals to ensure targets are met, but they can rush and be impatient with others, preferring to get on with things. They like to do things that can be implemented immediately, and are not for lengthy discussion. When teaching a pragmatist, you will need to set tasks and give them cases or projects to work on. Like the others, they can also be motivated by having to write up and report back upon their findings.

Thinking about the different approaches

If you wanted to teach a student how to take a person's blood pressure, how would you do this if they were a . . .

- Reflector?

- Activist?

- Theorist?

- Pragmatist?

Think about yourself in relation to your learning. Do you like to:

- Apply ideas in practice (pragmatist)?

- Observe and reflect (reflector)?

- Experience and do (activist)?

- Think and conceptualise (theorist)?

Do one or more of these suit you?

Visual-audio-kinaesthetic (VAK) model

This model suggests that there are three types of learner: visual, auditory, and kinaesthetic.

Visual learners learn through seeing and reading. These learners are said to need to see the teacher's body language, gestures, and facial expressions. They position themselves near the teacher in order to see better. They are said to think in pictures and be especially receptive to visual images, diagrams, displays, demonstrations, and films, etc. They often prefer to write things down and take detailed notes.

Auditory learners learn through hearing and talking. These learners prefer verbal lessons, listening to others, and talking things through or reciting facts. They are said to listen carefully, picking up on tone and pitch of the voice and searching for underlying implications. They need to hear things and often benefit from reading out loud and recording lectures.

Kinaesthetic learners learn through doing. These are active, tactile people who learn best with and prefer a hands-on approach, trying things out physically. They find it hard to sit for long periods and prefer to actively explore.

Again, as with Kolb and Honey and Mumford, we might have a preferred style but are capable of adapting and switching to others as the situation demands. If we know what a learner's preference is, we can then adapt our teaching methods to account for this. In a large group, it is thus good practice to vary the methods of teaching to involve something from each of the three categories. By doing this you will also be helping learners to explore new approaches to learning.

Try it online

Search for 'learning styles' online and you will find a range of tools for testing what learning style you have in relation to VAK and Kolb. Try them and see if you agree.

Criticisms of learning styles

Not everyone is convinced about the existence or value of learning styles and there is a degree of scepticism about the research. Many regard their claims as exaggerated (Tennant 1997) and over-simplistic. Coffield *et al.* (2004), for example, found no fewer than 71 different theories of learning styles, and pointed out that few of them were validated by independent research; they were rather scathing, suggesting that many theories make 'overblown' claims and that we place 'unwarranted faith in simple inventories'. The authors believe we should use our common sense instead. Coffield and colleagues argue that it is obvious different learners have different ways of learning, and that it is also obvious that teachers should use a variety of teaching methods to account for this. Another criticism is that learning styles are not necessarily fixed and can be chosen according to circumstance. Thus the learner chooses to learn in slightly different ways according to the task they are set and material they are trying to learn, so that we each have a mix of varying styles we can use.

Implications for teaching

There are many theories and opinions, but few hard facts. However, each theory gives us a different way of looking at and interpreting learning and what we experience, and that itself is a positive. We can also draw out of the debate some guidance for best practice.

For teachers and mentors, the implication is that learners will learn best when information is taught in a way that suits their preferred learning style. Some students will want to see the practical application first and then look at the theory behind it (pragmatists), while others will want to know everything about it first before they are willing to try it out in practice (theorists). Teachers need to be aware that there will likely be a range of learning styles in any group of students. For Kolb, learning is enhanced the more stages of the cycle the learner passes through and thus we should encourage learners to engage with all four stages, as each stage is a different way of learning.

To help find out about a student's preferred learning style, you should have a general discussion about their previous learning experiences, both negative and positive. Ask the student to list what helped them to learn and what hindered them. You can also use Kolb's stages to explore the mode of learning they like best and get them to think about the different learning styles and where they think they fit in. This will help them to expand and develop their repertoire and receptivity to different approaches to learning.

Remember that it is a good learning experience to take people out of their comfort zones every now and again (S. Hepworth, personal communication, 2009).

Because of the diversity of styles and stages, teachers need to develop a range of methods to cater for these. Repetition is an essential part of learning and if teaching repeats the same message via different methods geared to different styles or stages, it will likely be more effective.

Bloom's taxonomy, learning objectives, and competencies

Bloom (1956) attempted to classify all learning into three domains: cognitive, psychomotor, and affective – these are often referred to as 'head', 'hands', and 'heart' respectively. Bloom's work is especially important for vocational and professional training. It is relevant for nursing in particular, as it lends itself to the unique blend of knowledge, skills, and underpinning attitude that pervades all aspects of nursing care. Bloom is not describing learning styles but helping us to distinguish levels of learning so that we might logically progress from being a novice to being competent. In this way, it is easy to see the link between it and the progression of a student nurse throughout their training; indeed, many nursing curricula are guided by Bloom's taxonomy.

Bloom's domains

Cognitive	Head	Intellectual ability/knowledge
Psychomotor	Hands	Manual dexterity skills
Affective	Heart	Attitudes and values

Bloom's taxonomy is a classification of learning objectives (see Figure 4.5). Each domain is organised as a series of levels. Within each domain, it is suggested that the lowest level should be achieved before higher levels are addressed. The taxonomy therefore provides a sequential model for organising topics in the curriculum. This fits with the cognitive theory of

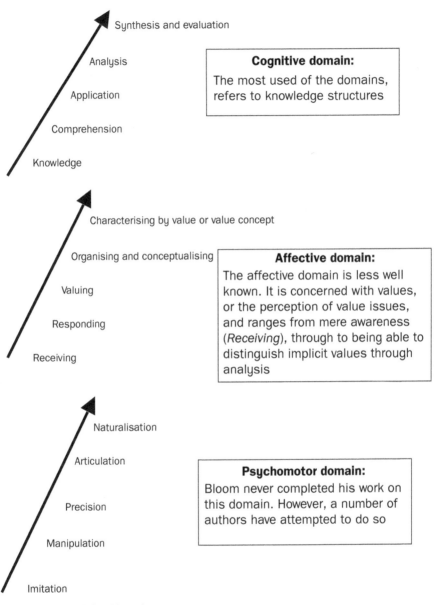

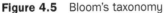

Figure 4.5 Bloom's taxonomy

Bruner with respect to logical sequencing, and that of Ausubel with respect to building upon existing knowledge. It also suggests a way of categorising levels of learning and defining the level of the expected outcomes. For example, in the cognitive domain, training for technicians or support workers may cover knowledge, comprehension, and application, whereas professional training may be expected to include this as well as synthesis and evaluation.

Cognitive domain (head)

This domain relates to intellectual abilities, thought processes, and the acquisition of knowledge.

Levels within the cognitive domain

- Knowledge   Recalling information and facts
- Comprehension   Understanding its meaning, interpreting it
- Application   Putting it into practice
- Analysis   Examining its structure, elements, and their interrelationships
- Synthesis   Using it and creating your own variation or adaptation
- Evaluation   Measuring its effectiveness

Psychomotor domain (hands)

This domain relates to motor skills, dexterity, and hand-to-eye coordination – practical skills.

Levels within the psycho-motor domain

- Imitation   Having a go, copying and trying it out under guidance
- Manipulation   Performing from memory
- Precision   Performing reliably and independently
- Articulation   Combining and integrating several skills
- Naturalisation   Demonstrating mastery

Affective domain (heart)

This domain relates to values, beliefs, attitudes, and ethics – emotions and feelings.

Levels within the affective domain

- Receive   Awareness of issues

- Respond   Able to discuss issues

- Value   Exploring other ideas, forming preferences, and becoming critical

- Organise   Organises beliefs and values

- Characterise   Internalises values and ideas

What domains would this teaching be aimed at?

- Aseptic technique

- A discussion around consent to treatment under the Mental Health Act

- Communication skills

- Giving an intramuscular injection

- Breaking bad news

- CPR

It is clear that whatever we teach, one domain will be dominant, but it is equally clear that whatever we teach will relate to elements of all three domains.

The domains are also very useful for lesson planning, helping to ensure each aspect is covered.

Think of a teaching session you might do with students:

- How will you cover the three domains?

- How will you assess the learning for each domain?

Out of the work of Bloom and others comes the idea of work-based competencies centred on knowledge, skills, and attitudes. These are arranged into levels to create a framework for their acquisition. Such competency-based taxonomies are used in much professional education and the NMC's (2010) *Standards for Pre-registration Nursing Education*. Students work through a series of levels of competence as they progress through the curriculum.

Student and mentor reflections

Student – the importance of repetition and an understanding mentor

I don't know what it was but I just couldn't get taking a BP right. We'd done it to death at uni, and most of my friends in our cohort could do it, so I felt it was becoming a big thing for me. I felt as though I would never get it right. My mentor was great – she made it sound that it was not a big deal and explained that she too had struggled with some procedures. She somehow took the pressure off and relaxed me about it. She said the best way to learn was to try and teach someone else. So she made me take a 'sphyg' home and practise on my partner. She said I had to explain to him how it worked and what everything was and what the readings meant. She made me take hers every shift and she'd take mine too, and I think it was this constant repetition that finally got me over the hurdle.

Mentor – self-awareness

I've had lots of first years, even second years and some thirds who got really worked up over things like their first injection or not being able to do a procedure, especially when most of the others around them were doing it. When you have been doing it for years, it's easy to get a bit frustrated yourself and think, 'On come on'. But then I have to just give myself a reminder of what I was like when I trained and how long it took me to grasp what to the nurses was a simple basic task. Now I go out of my way to be patient and just reassure them that they will get there in the end and that it's not a race.

Mentor – anxiety affects learning

Because we work with anxious people, we ought to be better able to recognise it in our students. Everyone who is in hospital is anxious to a degree, and we often overlook this to the detriment of their recovery. It's the same with the students. In mental health, we are often in counselling situations and I always remember what I learnt in my counselling training. The tutor used to ask us, 'What's on top?' He meant us to think about what was uppermost in our minds, because if we can't stop thinking about it we can't give our clients our attention. It's the same with students – you need to find what's on top for them. If there is something bothering them, either personal or professional and they can't get it out of their heads, then they can't learn or give things their best attention. We have to remember that students are real people too.

(continued)

Mentor – variety is the spice of life

It's not rocket science but a bit of behavioural theory goes a long way, especially in getting a student to grips with something that they are struggling with. The more you repeat something, the more you remember it and master it. On top of this, if you vary the ways you repeat something, it becomes more interesting and sinks in even further. Some like to watch, some like to read, and some like to do, but its best if they do all. So I'll give them a mix of practice – reading, discussion, and observation – and try and get them to teach others. They get there in the end.

Student – daunting but inspiring role modelling

I have to admit I was initially taken aback at just how professional they were in the team. There was a good laid-back atmosphere, but it didn't get in the way. They had very high standards and as a result had very high expectations of me. What was good was that they made it very clear as to what they expected, so I was in no doubt and they gave me realistic tasks but expected me to do them to a high standard. Because they respected me and had faith in my ability to live up to their expectations, it spurred me on and rubbed off on me. In many respects, they were doing with me what they did with the clients they were helping. I learnt that a lot of respect comes from being that skilled and professional and that it's important to have faith in people and give clear and realistic expectations and the support to reach them.

Summary of key principles of good teaching

- Student and teacher treat each other as equals.
- There should be a safe environment and a non-judgemental, welcoming atmosphere.
- The student needs to be motivated.
- Anxiety affects learning.
- Teaching should be student centred.
- The environment should be conducive to learning.
- The teacher must be approachable.
- The teacher facilitates and provides resources and opportunities.
- Teaching encompasses all of Kolb's stages of learning.
- Teaching should use a wide variety of methods and techniques.

- Problem-solving and experiential learning are effective.
- Reflection on learning and action is important.
- Students should be exposed to a wide range of experiences.
- Teaching recognises students' individuality and learning style.
- The teacher helps the student to accept responsibility for their own learning.
- Repetition is important.
- Positive reinforcement is useful and more effective than negative rein-forcement.
- Praise and reinforcement should be close to the event.
- Role modelling can exert a powerful influence.
- Learning should be active, not passive.
- Many people learn by 'doing'.
- Goal-setting can be an important motivator.
- Learning should match the learner's pace and ability.
- Learning should be practised.
- Learning should be pleasurable.
- Learning should be presented in a logical sequence.
- Learning should build upon what the learner already knows and their past experience.
- It's important for learners to see the big picture or where the learning fits in.
- Learners often need to see the practical application of theory.
- High expectations often yield high achievement.
- For all learning there are head, hands, and heart elements.

Summary

This chapter has:

- Examined behaviourist, cognitive, and humanistic educational theories
- Explored the concept of learning styles
- Discussed how Bloom's taxonomy is particularly useful in the nursing context for setting learning objectives
- Summarised the key principles of good teaching

Having examined the theory of teaching, it is pertinent to explore the application of that theory in practice. This is the focus of the next chapter, 'Teaching in practice'.

Further reading

Dix, G. and Hughes, S.J. (2004) Strategies to help students learn effectively, *Nursing Standard*, 18(32): 39–42.

Gopee, N. (2008) *Mentoring and Supervision in Healthcare*. London: Sage. This is an excellent book. Chapter 2, 'How learners learn' and Chapter 3, 'Facilitating learning' complement this chapter.

Honey, P. and Mumford, A. (1992) *The Manual of Learning Styles*, 3rd edn. Maidenhead: Peter Honey. It is worth reading the original authors' views rather than the interpretations of others.

Kolb, D.A. and Fry, R. (1975) Towards an applied theory of experiential learning, in C. Cooper (ed.) *Theories of Group Process*. London: Wiley. As above, it is wise to read the original works and Kolb has been commented upon by many and often misinterpreted.

Race, P. (2005) *Making Learning Happen*. London: Sage. In Chapter 3, 'Beyond learning styles', Race offers an intelligent critique of learning styles and an examination of what helps us to learn.

Snelgrove, S. (2004) Approaches to learning of student nurses, *Nurse Education Today*, 24(8): 605–14.

References

Ausubel, D.P. (1968) *Educational Psychology: A cognitive view*. New York: Holt, Rinehart & Winston.

Ausubel, D. (1978) In defence of advance organisers: a reply to the critics, *Review of Educational Research*, 48: 251–7.

Bandura, A. (1977) *Social Learning Theory*. Englewood Cliffs, NJ: Prentice-Hall.

Benner, P. (1984) *From Novice to Expert: Excellence and power in clinical nursing practice*. Menlo Park, CA: Addison-Wesley.

Bloom, B.S. (1956) *Taxonomy of Educational Objectives, Handbook I: The cognitive domain*. New York: David McKay.

Bruner, J.S. (1966) *Towards a Theory of Instruction*. Cambridge, MA: Belknap Press.

Coffield, F., Moseley, D., Hall, E. and Ecclestone, K. (2004) *Should We be Using Learning Styles? What research has to say about practice*. London: Learning Skills Resource Centre.

Dewey, J. (1933) *How We Think*. New York: Heath.

Dewey, J. (1974) My pedagogic creed, in R. Archambault (ed.) *John Dewey on Education*. Chicago, IL: University of Chicago Press.

Gibbs, G. (1988) *Learning by Doing: A guide to teaching and learning methods*. Oxford: Further Education Unit, Oxford Brookes University.

Honey, P. and Mumford, A. (1988) Setting the scene for learning styles, in C.M. Downie and P. Bashford (eds.) *Teaching and Assessing in Clinical Practice*. London: University of Greenwich Press.

Knowles, M. (1990) *The Adult Learner: A neglected species*, 4th edn. Houston, TX: Gulf Publishing.

Kolb, D.A. (1984) *Experiential Learning: Experience as the source of learning and development*. Englewood Cliffs, NJ: Prentice-Hall.

Lewin, K. (1946) Action research and minority problems, *Journal of Social Issues*, 2(4): 34–46.

Maslow, A. (1987) *Motivation and Personality*, 3rd edn. New York: Harper & Row.

Nursing and Midwifery Council (NMC) (2008) *Standards to Support Learning and Assessment in Practice: NMC standards for mentors, practice teachers and teachers*, 2nd edn. London: NMC.

Nursing and Midwifery Council (NMC) (2010) *Standards for Pre-registration Nursing Education*. London: NMC. Available at: http://standards.nmc-uk.org/Published Documents/Standards%20for%20pre-registration%20nursing%20education%20 16082010.pdf [accessed 2 March 2014].

Skinner, B.F. (1938) *The Behaviour of Organisms*. New York: Appleton Century Crofts.

Tennant, M. (1997) *Psychology and Adult Learning*, 2nd edn. London: Routledge.

Teaching in practice

Leadership

- Provide feedback about the effectiveness of learning and assessment in practice

Reflection on teaching

Think back to a teaching session you have given, whether formal or informal.

- Did you prepare for it or plan it in any way?
- What resources did you use?
- Did you evaluate it?
- If you were to do it again, what would you do differently?

Such practical questions are the focus of this chapter.

Theory in practice!

Although much educational theory can at times seem distant from practice and of limited value, there are certain teaching 'truths' derived from theory that are worth bearing in mind. These truths suggest that people learn better when:

- they want to learn;
- they think the material is important;
- they believe it has practical relevance;
- they think it will make a difference;
- the learning environment is supportive and free from threats;
- the teaching is varied and information is presented in different ways;
- they can try it out and practise 'hands on';
- they are given feedback and praise;
- they have some peer support.

Retention of learning

The evidence also suggests that how information is conveyed and used has a direct bearing upon how much is retained. In general, people are said to remember:

(continued)

- 10% of what they read
- 20% of what they hear
- 30% of what they see
- 50% of what they see and hear
- 70% of what they discuss with others
- 80% of what they do and use in life
- 95% of what they teach others to do

There are two basic behavioural principles at play in the above lists, namely, repetition and reinforcement. When information is given in a variety of ways, it is being repeated and rehearsed and thus stands more chance of being embedded in long-term memory rather than being temporarily stored in short-term memory and subsequently forgotten.

First-year mental health student

It didn't make any sense at all until she actually showed me. Every time she tried to explain it, I just couldn't get my head around it, but as soon as I saw her do it, it just clicked.

Positive reinforcement via praise and encouragement also acts as a reminder of the importance of the learning and underpins its retention. Oliver and Endersby (2000) encapsulate this when they suggest that good teaching can be summed up as follows: 'tell them what you are going to tell them, tell them, and then remind them of what you have told them'.

Repetition and variety

Alongside praise, repetition is key to helping people learn. The best way of repeating your message is by doing so in a variety of ways. Think about a teaching session you give or would like to give. List the different ways in which you could get your message across.

Lesson planning

Although lesson planning is obvious, it is often ignored and an unplanned lesson often fails to meet the needs of the students. Lesson planning is another cycle strongly reminiscent of the nursing process (see Figure 5.1).

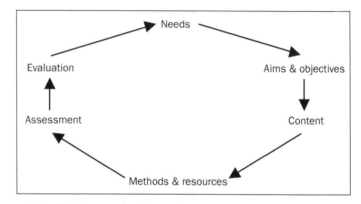

Figure 5.1   The lesson planning cycle

A carefully planned lesson should ensure that you don't miss anything crucial and that you logically sequence the material.

Teasdale (1993) argues that much clinical teaching is unstructured and often over-reliant on role modelling. The student works alongside a trained nurse and it is hoped they pick up good practice in the process. Teasdale suggests that mentors need to structure their teaching, arguing that there is a fundamental difference between practising nursing and teaching it, between demonstrating expertise and passing it on to others. One way of trying to ensure teaching occurs is using a teaching plan. Teaching plans should not be complicated; they should guide you in identifying the most important aspects of the session to be taught. The following is an example of a simple teaching plan that can be easily adapted for any teaching session.

Teaching plan

Subject

- Monitoring respirations

Aims

- Students will be able to accurately monitor respirations
- Students will be able to accurately record respirations

Objectives

- Explain normal respiration
- Explain common respiration variations and the reasons for such
- List the steps and techniques in the procedure
- Measure and record respirations

(continued)

Content
- Explanation of normal biology and reasons for and types of variation
- Explanation of procedure and correct ways of recording results

Method
- Lecture
- Demonstration
- Practice

Resources
- Respiration charts
- 'Do Not Disturb' sign for room

Handout
- Key points
- Correctly filled in respiration chart
- References and reading

Assessment
- Observation
- Question and answer

Evaluation
- Questionnaire

Factors to take into account

The needs of any session will be governed by several factors:

- The level of the student
- The NMC competencies
- The student's personal learning needs and interests
- The clinical area specialism
- The resources available
- Time

The students' learning needs will largely consist of the NMC competencies they have to achieve in that placement, but there may be particular objectives that the student wishes to concentrate upon. They may be keen to practise a certain procedure or find out about a particular aspect of care that is peculiar to that placement. The mentor will also have to take into account the level which any particular student is at. Are they an anxious first-year student with little previous healthcare experience, or a confident third-year student with a strong healthcare background? Assessing these needs and factors will be a prime focus of the initial meeting and first week of working with the student. This information will be important in guiding the focus and delivery of subsequent teaching sessions.

Newly qualified nurse tutor

I used to just think I had to tell them everything I knew about X, Y or Z, and I'd end up just talking at them for ages and giving them a huge handout. It was only when I started to really plan the sessions that I began to break the information down into manageable chunks. Actually writing the lesson plan out made it so much easier for me and the students got a more realistic session, better focused and more varied.

Aims and objectives

Warning! One of the biggest dangers in teaching is that of information overload, trying to cover too much material. A teaching session is always partly an introduction, after which the student should be inspired to go away and fill in the gaps in a bout of self-directed learning. In fact, a good teaching session can be likened to being given a jigsaw with a few pieces missing – the student then has to go away and find those pieces!

Having identified the students' learning needs, aims and objectives must be set for several important reasons:

- To keep the teaching focused on what is important
- To enable you to evaluate if the teaching session was effective or not
- To enable the students to understand what the prime focus is
- To define the content and what methods to use

The aim is a broad, general goal from which the more specific objectives derive. The aim should tell you what the student ought be able to do after the teaching session.

Example of aims and objectives

LESSON	Baked beans
AIM	To cook a tin of beans
OBJECTIVES	Identify the equipment needed
	Demonstrate safe tin opening
	Operate the cooker effectively to heat the beans through
	Present an edible serving

Objectives are the steps that need to be taken to achieve the aim and should be clearly written using the following guidelines. They can be regarded as learning outcomes and need to have the following two qualities:

1. Objectives should be stated using verbs that describe behaviour or actions. This is so that they can be observed and assessed.

2. Objectives should be SMART:

- **Specific**   small and/or logically sequenced
- **Measurable**   so as to be able to evaluate and assess
- **Achievable**   realistic for the level of the student
- **Relevant**   to the competencies and students' needs
- **Timed**   realistically achievable in the time available

Objectives and Bloom's taxonomy

The objectives can be written using Bloom's taxonomy as a guide and can be drawn from any of the three domains. Thus a good lesson plan will cover the cognitive, psychomotor, and affective aspects of any subject:

Cognitive	the knowledge base
Psychomotor	the hands-on, practical skills
Affective	the underpinning attitudes and values

Writing objectives will become easier with practice, so try the following exercise.

Exercise

Thinking about encompassing all three of Bloom's domains, write an overall aim and several (SMART) objectives for the following:

- Hand washing

- Monitoring respirations

- Gaining informed consent

It is also useful to refer to lists of words appropriate to each of the domains, such as those in the box below.

Useful words for writing objectives

Cognitive domain

Name, label, list, select, state, explain, demonstrate, show, justify, discriminate between, break down, categorise, create, judge, argue, compare, criticise, contrast, analyse, describe, give examples of, define, interpret, restate, propose

Psychomotor domain

Perform, repeat, arrange, identify, show, calculate, prepare, build, produce, chart, practise, measure, set up, demonstrate, adapt, alter, modify, combine, manage, design

Affective domain

Choose, acknowledge, select, identify, respond, justify, compare, challenge, evaluate, contrast, distinguish between, arrange, organise, modify, argue, defend, critique

---

Remember that in Bloom's taxonomy each domain has several levels of achievement, so ensure that the objectives are appropriate to the level of the lesson and learner.

Experienced nurse tutor

It's almost impossible to assess the sessions you give if you don't set clear objectives. If you are not specific in what you want to achieve, you cannot tell if you get there. You need to be quite basic: 'This is what I want the student to know', 'This is what I want the student to be able to do'.

Content

The content of a teaching session can also be derived by use of Bloom's taxonomy. The lesson should cover:

- knowledge, i.e. what the student needs to know;
- skills, i.e. what they need to do; and
- attitude, i.e. the manner in which it should be done.

While most subjects will encompass aspects of all three domains, certain subjects will be more related to one specific domain. For example, a session on ethical aspects of nursing will draw more heavily upon the affective domain, while one on aseptic technique will draw more heavily upon the psychomotor domain. Both, of course, will need to embrace the cognitive domain too.

Words of wisdom

Teasdale (1993) suggests that the content and lesson delivery can be easily broken into stages, such as explanation, demonstration, and practice. At each stage, the key points should be identified.

Ley (1988) demonstrated that when information is conveyed, the short-term memory is capable of remembering an average of only seven pieces of information. He also demonstrated that when a lot of information is being conveyed, people tend to forget what was in the middle and remember most the information they heard first and last.

Miller (1956) had earlier come to the same conclusions, arguing that most of us can take in no more than seven key pieces of information in any one teaching session.

What the above tells us, of course, is that we should limit the volume of information we convey to that which can be absorbed, and that if we have especially important things to say we should say them first or last. Emphasising key points along the way is also very important in reinforcing the message.

Learning contracts

Learning contracts are a useful aid to learning. These help students to learn on their own and are said to result in deeper learning because of the exploration undertaken by the learner as opposed to just being told or taught. In behavioural terms, such exploration of the material will also involve repetition and so the learning could be said to be more permanent. Learning contracts are also useful for fostering time management and self-directed learning skills.

A failing first-year student

I was very sceptical about the learning contract at first. It looked like a lot of work and I wasn't too keen but it really did focus me and make me concentrate on what I needed to do.

The learning contract is an agreement between the learner and their tutor or mentor that gives the learner structure and guidance for their learning. It begins with a mutual identification of the learner's learning needs and from that point it:

- sets objectives (what will be learnt);
- identifies resources;
- identifies methods and activities (reading, observation, etc.);
- sets goals with target times;
- identifies what constitutes evidence of achievement;
- is regularly reviewed.

The responsibility belongs to the student, who must plan and time-manage the contractual goals. The contract can be seen as an action plan outlining how the objectives will be met alongside an assessment strategy to test this. The assessment strategy should identify clearly what is to be assessed, by whom, how, and when.

Advantages and disadvantages of a learning contract

Advantages	Disadvantages
Students in an active role with regard to learning	Mentor and student can become worried about format
Increases motivation	Learners may have difficulty identifying learning needs
Responsibility rests with the student	Student may adopt a dependent role
Develops planning and self-management skills	Unrealistic goals may be set and this can result in anxiety
Helps to reconcile needs of student/education/employers	Can be time-consuming
Promotes self-assessment	Can restrict inventiveness
Promotes creativity	

Example of a learning contract

In the literature, you will find lots of good ways of setting out a learning contract. The following is an example for a student who has to meet a number of specified outcomes from their curriculum. The italic text in brackets is not part of the contract but serves to explain the thinking and rationale behind the contract.

LEARNING CONTRACT

Name of Learner: **Name of Mentor:**

INITIAL INTERVIEW SUMMARY: (*Record previous experience, special requirements, etc.*)

First Placement . . . .

(*This section should be completed adhering to the same standards that we apply to the recording of information about our patients/clients. For the purpose of this example, our learner is a first-year student nurse on their first clinical placement*)

IDENTIFIED LEARNING NEEDS/OBJECTIVES (please list):

To meet generic foundation skills 1a to i and 2a to g and 3a to c. See student's placement document for details.

(*There is no need to write out the outcomes if they are listed on other documents that form part of the student's record*)

LEARNING ACTION PLAN: (*What, who, when, and how*)

- Sylvia will show Sue where the relevant Trust policies and procedures are – Sue will read these during week 1 of the learning period.

- Sylvia will direct Sue to some relevant literature. Sue will locate and read other relevant literature professional guidelines and research summaries.

- Sylvia and Sue will discuss the above so that Sue can ask questions about anything that is not clear (weeks 1 and 2).

- Sylvia will explain and demonstrate the care activities included above on several occasions using routine care situations and some non-routine situations (week 1). We have agreed that Sue will work five shifts with Sylvia to enable this to take place.

- Sue will also observe other members of staff carrying out these aspects of care (week 1).

- Sue will attend a tutorial about . . . . (week 2).

- Sue will contribute to the care activities above under direct supervision and with the consent of patients/clients. On every occasion, Sue will agree with the supervising practitioner the care that she will undertake before doing so.

- During week 3 (if progress is confirmed and Sue is confident), Sue will (with patient/client consent) contribute to agreed activities with indirect supervision.

(*continued*)

RESOURCES:

(In this section, the relevant policies and procedures should be listed along with the references for any reading materials recommended and any personnel that may be able to help)

REVIEW ARRANGEMENTS: *(These should be mutually agreed in advance)*

ASSESSMENT PLAN:

'OUTCOME/S' TO BE ASSESSED:

Generic foundation skills 1a to i and 2a to g and 3a to c, as outlined in Sue's practice placement record.

CRITERIA FOR JUDGEMENT AND LEVEL REQUIRED: *(assessment tool)*

List of relevant Trust and professional body guidelines and/or research references – whatever sets the standard of care in these areas. Practice will be graded according to university grading criteria.

(Evidence-based assessment requires that the standard being used to assess is based on published professionally agreed criteria for good practice)

EVIDENCE REQUIRED: *(Assessment method/s, WHAT, WHEN, WHERE, WHO, AND HOW – time span)*

1 Performance – Amount and Type of Evidence:

We have agreed that:

- Sylvia (mentor) will observe Sue in all of the above activities over a period of at least ten working shifts – including observation of each separate activity on at least three separate occasions. Sylvia will specify the clients concerned at the start of the relevant shifts and agree with Sue the care activities that she will undertake.

- Sylvia will also ask RGN Jane to observe Sue (as above) with at least two clients during the assessment period. *(Strengthens the reliability of the decision – there is inter-rater agreement – reduces the risk of bias)*

- Sylvia will support Sue in self-assessment in relation to some aspect of each of the skill areas identified. *(This helps to reduce the risk of bias. It also engages the learner in the development of accountability and the self-regulation that forms part of the expectations of professional practice)*

(continued)

2 **Knowledge – Amount and Type of Evidence:**

Sylvia will ask Sue questions about:

- each of the activities carried out
- the Trust's policy/guidelines
- relevant professional body guidelines
- associated legal and ethical issues

Sylvia will also present a number of 'what if' scenarios for discussion (*Increases validity – makes sure that the knowledge demonstrated by the learner is not just rote learning*)

Any Special Arrangements Required:

Time-frame over which assessment will take place:

Five working days: –

Commence (*Date*)

Target Date for Completion:

No later than (*Date*)

Feedback and Review Arrangements:

REVIEW NOTES (continue over page as necessary):

RECORD OF OUTCOMES:

SIGNATURES and DATE:

Devised by Sylvia Hepworth, Principal Lecturer, University of Huddersfield.

There are many different learning contracts and it is good practice to adapt them and devise your own version to suit your particular situation or an individual student's needs. The following is a simplified version of a learning contract.

Learning contract

Name:

Learning outcomes to be met:

Resources and help required:

Activity to be undertaken (and by when):

Evidence of achievement:

Review date:

Signatures: Date:

Second-year adult field student

I had failed a few outcomes in a previous placement and I didn't get them because although I knew which competencies I had to get, I was never sure just how to get them or what I had to do and my mentor was quite vague. This time my mentor sat me down and we wrote out a plan of exactly what it was that I needed to do to achieve the ones I was missing.

Spontaneous teaching

There is no such thing as a planned curriculum for each placement; at best it is a list of possible learning experiences. Such structures as lesson planning, aims, objectives, and learning contracts are all well and good but as was mentioned in Chapter 3, much teaching on wards is of a spontaneous, seize-the-moment variety. As situations arise, they become learning opportunities and mentors turn action into teaching as it happens. Much clinical skills teaching takes place in this way, preceded or followed by more structured skills teaching.

Questions

- How might spontaneous practice experiences be turned into learning?

- How might you build in structured teaching or learning experiences in an otherwise busy and unpredictable environment?

Reflective discussions often underpin such spontaneous learning experiences and are useful in consolidating the learning to be drawn from these experiences. Alternatively, ask the student to write a reflective account of the experience and examine the evidence underpinning it. Spontaneous learning is often the case with skills whereby in an intensive burst of activity in a short time-frame, a student can often witness and be involved in a vast array of skills well delivered in difficult circumstances. The learning opportunities in such a scenario are legion. Imagine a 'crash' scenario and the practical, communication, and managerial skills involved. Or, a community psychiatric nurse encountering a client with clear suicidal intent. A good mentor must use such experiences to direct the student to explore and unpick them and then relate them to their competencies.

First year student on medical emergency assessment unit

It was all very quick . . . It was over before I knew it. A patient crashed quite unexpectedly. One moment there was panic (from me) and the

(continued)

next there was this completely professional, calm, assured process kicking in. It was very impressive and inspirational. My mentor just said be ready to help and watch. I was asked (something miniscule) but to me at the time such a big thing. Afterwards my mentor asked me to talk about what had happened and asked me if I could see anything that could have been done better (me!). He then asked me to write a reflection around the event and asked me to list the practical, management, and human skills involved in the scenario. It took me ages to write it all down because when I analysed it, there was so much and it only lasted 20 minutes.

Teaching methods and strategies

There will be certain methods that you prefer to use and feel better at delivering, but remember that you should also consider what is best for the student, given their learning style and which method is best for the material you are teaching.

Lectures

Lectures get information across directly and in a logical sequence and get large amounts of information across in a short time. They are more influential if delivered by a clinician or expert with current experience upon which to draw and who can relate the theory to practice examples. However, communication can be 'one way' and the audience can be left largely passive. It is good practice to allow a period for questions and answers at the end if not invited throughout. A lecture needs a time limit to be effective, as concentration tends to lapse beyond 40 minutes. Thus it needs variety and exercises in order to keep the students interested. Lectures reflect a cognitive approach to teaching in that they focus upon delivery of information that has then to be processed by the learner and memorised before it can be used. Evidence suggests that if we don't process or use the lecture information soon, the bulk of it quickly gets forgotten. Lectures are also a form of pedagogical teaching whereby the teacher informs the learner what they need to know.

Expert panels

Having experts on hand brings currency and credibility to a session, but it may be hard to organise and experts are not necessarily good teachers. However, their clinical credibility tends to make people listen. A panel can allow a useful dialogue and discussion of a range of opinions, especially if there is more than one expert. It is a great opportunity for open questions.

Critical incident analysis

This is an in-depth form of reflection. An incident (which, despite the name, does not have to be critical) is presented for discussion and group work. It may be a scenario or an example of practice, either good or bad. Critical incident analysis usually:

- describes the incident in some detail;
- gives its context;
- explains why it was important to you;
- describes your initial and subsequent thoughts and feelings and actions;
- identifies issues and dilemmas;
- examines what helped and what hindered;
- tries to look at alternative ways of seeing the incident;
- looks at what you might do differently next time.

Thus, a critical incident analysis represents a useful way of examining practice and aiding personal and professional development. Students can be encouraged to use this structure or method and to present a critical analysis of something they have experienced and wish to examine in more depth. Also, note the similarity to the action research process. Critical incident analysis pays homage to Bruner's (1966) assertion that teaching should be focused upon problem-solving. Such an analysis also relies heavily upon the work of Kolb and others in relation to the importance of reflection.

Reflective practice sessions

In such sessions, students are primed to bring along an incident or situation or client problem and discuss their reflection of it and open up a debate with the others present.

Reflective diaries/writing

These are personal learning documents that can be drawn upon to identify learning needs and provide a focus for discussion with mentors. They are developmental in that they allow the writer to chart and reflect upon their progress through an experience.

Role-play/experiential exercises

A role-play adds much needed variety to learning, but some students find it threatening so they must be properly prepared. It gives the players the chance to experience how others might feel and to see problems in a different light (i.e. as others might see it). It is also a good opportunity to practise communication and other skills. Videotaping the role-play can add another dimension, providing a unique opportunity for analysing skills and gaining some self-awareness. We rarely get the opportunity to see ourselves in a professional role. To be most effective, it needs to be done with small groups and the groups need to be warned in advance and not just sprung on them.

Another frequent use of role-play is to gain an understanding of the perspective of others, such as patients. Students can take on the role of patients in a variety of settings, such as being interviewed or having blood pressure taken. The discussion following the role-play is crucial for drawing out the learning from the experience.

Other useful experiential learning exercises include such simple experiences as sitting in an outpatient department for an hour and trying to get around in a wheelchair. Mentors could be quite creative here. Mental health nursing students could experience a period of seclusion, and any student who is lucky enough to never have spent a night in hospital should be invited to do so in a hospital bed and perhaps lay there all day without visitors and share the patients' meals and timetable. One creative nurse tutor I knew had her students wear a colostomy bag full of Weetabix for a day. Whether role-playing or undertaking experiential exercises, it is important that everyone is de-roled and allowed to discuss the experience in some depth, as it can often raise emotional responses in participants.

Second-year student mental health nurse

I didn't go in that day. I hate being video'd and role-playing. It makes me nervous. Two other people in the group refused to do it as well.

Second-year student mental health nurse

It was really quite interesting to see yourself in that way. You don't often get to see yourself in 'work' mode and I was amazed at just how I came across. I had no idea I fidgeted so much.

Role-play draws some of its rationale from cognitive theory and reflects the importance of experiential learning theory.

Workshops

These can be a blend of theory input and skills practice and be open to a wide range of people. They are heavily interactive, encourage participation, and draw upon discussion and the experience of the participants, as well as the skills of experts. They are also an opportunity to move from the classroom back into the practice area. Holding the workshops on the ward or in the clinic can allow them to become open to all, so that staff, clients, and others can drop in and participate.

Group discussions

A group discussion needs a stimulating focus or trigger and a facilitator to get it up and running and to keep it focused. The facilitator needs to ensure that everyone is involved, and that it is not dominated by a vocal minority. It also needs a relatively small group to encourage wide participation. Group discussion is a good way of encouraging reflection, providing feedback, and motivating students. Group discussion needs to heed the wisdom of human-istic approaches to teaching by ensuring that the atmosphere is welcoming, democratic, and inclusive. Such discussions are also an expression of the andragogical principle, which respects the views of the learner.

Seminars/literature reviews/journal clubs

These entail a presentation and discussion, often examining a recent article or examining the literature surrounding a certain topic. It may be that each week a student is asked to review an article from a journal relevant to the clinical area. These sessions need not be long and can be quite informal. They will be enhanced if the article is circulated before the session; in this way, everyone will be familiar with the material and in a better position to comment.

Evidence-based practice

Evidence-based practice is at the heart of the above teaching methods and strategies. It is easy for mentors to assume that students are aware of the evidence behind what they do, especially if they appear competent. It does no harm to clarify this by asking the student to present it. This also acts as a valuable updating tool for the mentor, who can appraise their view in the light of what might be fresh evidence from the student. It is a very positive way of sharing. The mentor can choose any task or proce-dure and ask the student to appraise the evidence base behind it. Another good approach is to look at the NICE guidelines and critique them in the light of the student's and mentor's practice experience. If there is a con-flict, the question arises as to how can this be fed into the evidence pool. See the section on Action Research in Chapter 3.

Question-and-answer sessions

A student-focused question-and-answer session is a simple and effective way of allowing students to drive the focus of a session and direct it to their own particular learning needs. Students bring questions to the group for the group to answer collectively. One good variation upon this is for each student to bring a written question for the group. These are then folded and redistributed so that each student gets someone else's question, which they try to answer before throwing it open to the group.

Mind storming

This can be a very creative way of generating a range of ideas for discussion and points of view or solutions. It is a good way of starting a session and getting things going. If all responses are appreciated, it can be very inclusive and draw responses from the quieter members of the group. Ideas are generated from other ideas. Mind storming is good for building up a sense of group togetherness and can be fun, since 'offbeat' ideas are also encouraged because they often lead to more robust variations. It needs a good facilitator to get it going and bring it back together. Ensure that all responses are written down on a flipchart to refer back to.

Concept/mind maps

These are a way of exploring and expanding a subject and breaking it down into its parts. Variations are sometimes called 'spider charts' or 'tree diagrams'. A main subject is placed in the centre from which lines extend out to identify its constituent parts, as in the 'Role of the nurse' spider chart in Figure 3.1. Then lines are extended from these outer entities, breaking them down into their parts. There will also be some cross-referencing between parts, and there can be many branches and sub-branches. It can get quite complicated and messy but it is a useful way of exploring a subject, since putting pen to paper somehow helps you to see it from a wider perspective and appreciate interrelationships that were not previously apparent. It is a useful way of getting a group of students to explore an issue, especially if they can do it on flipchart paper or a big whiteboard (see Figure 5.2).

Case study/conference

A case study session or case conference is good for exploring many aspects of care. It will foster a problem-solving approach and engage the students at many levels (e.g. clinical skills, management, education, attitude). A case study is good at generating a range of ideas and is itself a good problem-solving tool when applied to difficult patient scenarios or difficult clinical problems. It can highlight areas for further learning. A key feature of a case study is that it often provides the opportunity to relate the theory to practice and real life. Another key feature of case studies is that they tend to foster an appreciation of the roles of other members of the multidisciplinary team. When the outcome of an analysis of a care plan review or case

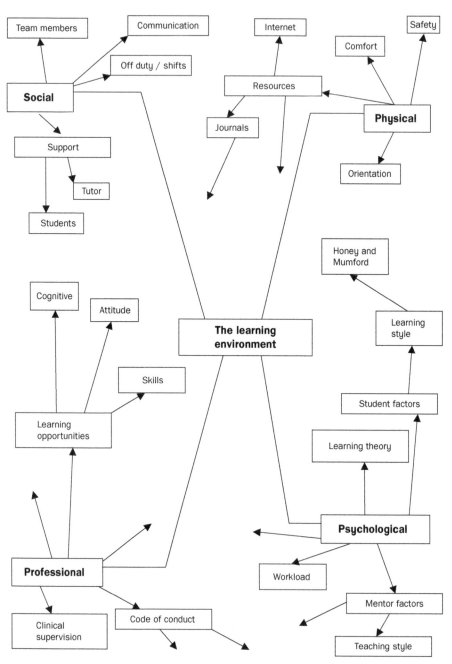

Figure 5.2   Example of the construction of a mind map

study is given as a presentation to the team, it is another good opportunity for the student to develop and practise other key skills such as team working and teaching.

Third-year mental health student

It was a very good experience to attend the conference with so many qualified nurses. My mentor was presenting and she took me along. It made me feel I was part of the profession. To be invited was good in itself – it showed that they valued the contribution of students, and I learnt so much more than I could have done by just reading around the subject.

Role modelling

A competent, safe, evidence-based mentor is perhaps the best teaching tool, as students will hold them in high esteem and learn from them almost by osmosis. 'Sitting by Nellie' was the old term for this, as apprentices just sat and watched the master at work in order to pick up their skills. It is a form of behaviourist social learning (Bandura 1977) whereby we watch others we hold in high regard perform and see the positive outcomes of their actions and so wish to mimic their behaviour in order to achieve the same outcomes. This is arguably how most learning occurs on placements; unfortunately, it is also how bad practice can be easily picked up, underlining the need for mentors to use evidence-based practice and have a positive outlook. This is important because it is not just knowledge and skills that students pick up from role models, but attitudes as well. If the 'real' learning in nursing occurs in the workplace, and much of that learning occurs via role modelling, the importance of the role of the mentor and the need for highly skilled and highly professional mentors becomes evident.

Task-setting

A bit like homework, task-setting gives people the opportunity to go and find things out for themselves and then report back. It can allow students to work at their own pace and set their own agenda, or be directed by the mentor. Individuals or groups of students can be given small projects to complete during their placement. These can be linked to the student outcomes and competencies so as to provide evidence of achievement.

Exercises/quizzes

Quizzes speak for themselves and are relatively easy to devise. Specific exercises for students can be much more intricate but a good mentor can devise many good learning exercises for students to undertake and relate them to the NMC outcomes and competencies the students have to achieve.

The following is an example of a case study for first-year mental health field students that can be easily adapted for all fields.

First-year student case study exercise

In collaboration with your mentor, identify a service user who may be willing for you to undertake a case study of their care needs and care plan.

Gain consent from the service user and document how you obtained it.

Obtain the service user's views of their mental health problems and care needs. Identify the details of this interaction:

- How did you start the conversation?

- What helped or hindered your engagement with the client?

- What do you understand by the term 'effective communication'?

- What does the literature say?

Read the service user's notes and plan of care. Consider the following:

- Does it reflect the service user's view of their problems and care needs?

- If there are differences, why could these be?

- What assessment tools were used?

- What is the rationale for the planned care?

- What national and local policies guide the care given?

- Is the plan holistic and what does this mean?

Map these to the NMC pre-registration domains and competencies and to the 'Code'.

(Devised by Fran Maplethorpe)

If the above case study was subsequently presented to the team, it would enable the student to achieve more outcomes.

Task: exercises

Exercises reflect the cognitive theory of Ausubel (1978), in that they build upon prior knowledge. We give the student a piece of information and ask them to perform an exercise that leads to further learning or consolidation. Many such exercises relate to the testing out of theory in practice.

(continued)

What other exercises might you be able to construct relevant to your clinical area that will help towards the student's achievement of the NMC competencies?

The Internet

The Internet is an invaluable tool because of its ability to provide us with wide-ranging and up-to-date information, and students can be asked to research aspects of practice to report back to the team. However, beware the student who hides behind the computer and who is more assignment-focused than placement-focused. If this happens, the mentor needs to find out the underlying reasons, offer support, and key the student back into the placement.

Videos/DVDs

These provide variety and present information visually as well as verbally. They keep the group's attention unless they are too long and wander off the point. It is sometimes best to show short clips as a focus for group work or discussion rather than the whole recording. They require a good facilitator to set the scene and generate responses and guide group work afterwards.

Handouts

In his work on communication, Ley (1988) reminds us that memory fades over time and that it is important to give written back-up. The ethos of evidence-based practice demands that any handouts are fully referenced.

Visits to other departments/working with other members of the multidisciplinary team

Many opportunities will arise for students to undertake insight visits to other areas connected with the clinical area they are placed in. These may not necessarily be nursing/medical, and can often be social services or voluntary agencies that play a part in patient support and aftercare. There are also many allied professions with whom we work and days spent with these can provide an invaluable insight into their respective roles and a better understanding of the workings and importance of the multidisciplinary team. From the consultant psychiatrist to the hospital chaplain or pharmacist, there will be many opportunities in any one clinical area.

Talking to patients and relatives

Although patients are a learning resource, we tend to underuse them and their families in nurse education. We ultimately practise procedures and communication skills on and with patients, but how frequently do we encourage the students to sit and talk with them to get an insight into the human side of being away from home, being scared, and feeling lonely? Students should be encouraged to audit the client experience via such conversations so that they can keep in touch with the patient experience and help ensure humanistic rather than mechanistic care. It is easy for students to lose this important perspective when they are being taught technical procedures and theories and are focused upon outcomes and competencies.

Resource area

Most clinical areas should also have a resource area for students as described in Chapter 3, 'The clinical learning environment'. This will include such teaching aids as equipment, flipcharts, books, journals, models, posters, policies, and leaflets.

Evidence-based practice

The following are ways to encourage students to engage with evidence-based practice:

- Ask the student to identify the different sources of evidence for the specialty.

- Ask the student to identify the different levels of evidence.

- Ask the student to look up policies and national guidelines for the specialty.

- Ask the student to research and present an evidence-based article.

- Ask the student to develop a comprehensive list of online resources for the clinical area.

- Ask the student to explore an area of care using relevant databases.

- Ask the student to reflect upon the professional and ethical implications of not using evidence-based practice.

Staff

The most important resources in any clinical setting are, of course, the staff. All clinical areas offer experiences but not all offer learning experiences – it is the mentors who make this difference.

Exercise: Evidence-based practice

For each of the teaching methods and strategies outlined above, identify the underpinning educational theory that supports them. Identify the key principles that govern how and why they work. Also consider which learning style such methods might appeal to.

Practical clinical skills teaching

Demonstration and practice is a mainstay of clinical skills teaching and to be effective it needs to be carried out in quite small groups to ensure that each participant is given sufficient attention. It is unsafe practice to try to teach a key skill to a large group. It is also crucial that the demonstrator can show the evidence base for the skill. Demonstration and practice is clearly a form of behavioural teaching whereby repetition leads to learning. It also relates to the ideas of Dewey (1974), who suggested that learning is best when it is active and practical. However, as we have already identified, most skills teaching occurs in practice by seizing upon opportunities as they arise throughout the working day. Skilled mentors turn their interventions into skills teaching sessions and follow these up with further explanation and practice. A good way of consolidating this is to arrange for students to teach skills to junior students while the mentor assesses them. The theory suggests we retain 95% of what we teach others and this is because in preparing the taught session we have to interact with the information to a deeper level. The following are some guidelines.

Principles for teaching one-to-one and in small groups

(a) Initial introductions and setting the scene

In teaching clinical skills, explaining your qualifications and experience and demonstrating how you maintain your skills are important if you are to retain the interest and motivation of your students. Share some pertinent details of your professional background, past and current experiences, and encourage your students to do the same. Personal anecdotes about when you learnt a particular procedure are usually well received and form an integral part of the culture of shared experience within nursing.

Adult learners are most receptive when they have a real and pressing need to learn a particular skill or procedure, as for example, in preparation for a practical assessment or before going out into clinical practice with their mentor. Help the student(s) to understand the relevance of the planned session by agreeing some simple learning objectives, placing

(continued)

the procedure into its clinical context, and 'signposting' the main theoretical perspectives (Fry et al. 2003).

(b) Value the prior experience of adult learners

It might seem self-evident, but it is essential to identify the relevant previous experiences and the level of knowledge of the individual learners before you start (Dix and Hughes 2005). Student nurses often have prior experience in health or social care, so if, for example, your session for first-year students focuses on the skills associated with urinalysis, identify those who might have learnt this procedure as part of a previous role. Acknowledging skills and knowledge indicates that you value their 'real-world' experience. It is useful to continue your dialogue with those students by actively seeking their perceptions from time to time: 'Was this a particular issue where you worked?'

(c) Establish a supportive learning environment

Teaching clinical skills is best performed in small groups, so initial, positive interactions between members will be instrumental in laying the foundations for the social learning to come. Such interactions facilitate metacognitive learning, as students closely identify with the opinions and views of colleagues and friends within their peer group (Biggs 1999).

Working in small groups helps students to develop transferable skills associated with team working in clinical practice, as the students actively collaborate in order to achieve an agreed outcome – in this case, competency in a particular procedure or technique. This involves negotiating turns in practising, providing feedback on their own and on their peers' performance, and demonstrating effective communication.

(d) Encourage ownership of procedure

It is advisable to provide the students with the evidence-based technique or procedure, split into stages in order for the students to better remember the steps involved. The stages should not be too detailed because, paradoxically, if you provide too much detail, it can over-complicate rather than simplify!

The procedure should always promote the personhood of the individual patient/client, for example by including the requirement to seek and document consent and to maintain dignity and privacy, in order to reduce the risk of students adopting a 'task-orientated' rather than patient-centred approach.

Practical techniques are usually demonstrated before the student practises under supervision. The demonstrator needs to be competent and confident in both the technique and their underpinning knowledge in

(continued)

order to provide a meaningful commentary in relation to the rationale and evidence base for each stage.

Students should then practise and familiarise themselves with the procedure through repetition.

Encourage them to rewrite the procedure, devising their own personal stages and prompts. This is particularly useful when preparing for a practical assessment, as the student can use it to aid their own memory via the 'silent-run through' or 'internal commentary technique' (Eason et al. 2012).

(e) Consider the use of simulation

Simulation is increasingly used within nurse education, as it represents a way in which students can practise their developing skills in a realistic setting without risk of harm to patients (Haidar 2009; Lewis and Ciak 2011). It is also an effective method of ensuring that all students obtain the specific clinical experiences required to meet their learning objectives (Larew et al. 2006).

Teaching students to change a simple dressing on a manikin using aseptic technique, for example, represents a low-fidelity but effective simulation. It has the advantage of allowing spontaneity when unexpected issues occur, such as when a student drops 'soiled' gauze onto the floor or pulls a hole in a sterile glove. As the patient within this scenario is not at risk, the group can focus on the range of options available to recover the situation, thereby promoting a problem-solving approach. Exploring issues in the immediacy of the moment helps to avoid students learning a procedure merely 'by rote' by promoting reflection and critical thinking.

(f) Expert versus peer teaching

As mentioned elsewhere in this book, experts are not always the best teachers. Arguably, this has a particular relevance in relation to practical, psychomotor skills. Sometimes the expert becomes so adept at performing a particular technique that they find it difficult to revisit the basics. Competent senior students have more recently learned, so might empathise more readily and have the patience required to take the student through the steps in a logical, unhurried way. Appropriate involvement in peer teaching also benefits the senior students, helping them to develop and to consolidate their own teaching skills (Stables 2012).

Summary of main points

- Facilitate introductions, share professional background and some insights of learning procedure

- Explain the relevance of the particular procedure and make explicit connections with clinical practice and associated theory

(continued)

- Identify and acknowledge the prior experience of individual learners

- Ensure the procedure used is patient-centred and evidence-based

- Break the procedure down into manageable stages

- Consider who is best placed to demonstrate and to answer student questions

- Encourage students to personalise the procedure and develop their own 'internal commentary'

- Provide opportunities for safe, repetitive practise and consider possible untoward events

- Allow time for reflection and for students to make own connections with pre-existing knowledge

- Signpost students to further sources of evidence-based information, including online resources

(Devised by Diane Ramm, Senior Lecturer,
University of Lincoln)

Presentations

The clinical area might have access to a computer with a PowerPoint presentation facility. These can be good teaching aids if used in moderation, but all too often a PowerPoint presentation is either too long or too crowded. A good PowerPoint presentation has few words on each slide around which the presenter can speak. It also uses graphics to stimulate and maintain interest. It should not be too long or consist of too many slides, as this becomes tedious after a while and students will lose interest (see Figures 5.3, 5.4, and 5.5). A presentation will need to be broken up with activity if it is to go on for any length of time.

Whether using PowerPoint or not, a good presentation will be characterised by the following:

- Presenter is confident and knowledgeable

- Clear aims and objectives are identified

- Presentation is pitched at level of learners

- There is an interesting introduction

- Presenter makes people feel at ease

- Material is logically sequenced

- Complex information is broken down

- Relevance to practice is apparent and examples cited

PowerPoint tips

~ Don't make the font too fancy

~ Use a clear font such as this, Arial or verdana

~ Don't make it too small ....Not less than 18 point

~ Or Too big

~ Take care with colours (red on blue for example is virtually impossible to read) and
  be aware that some forms of dyslexia will make it hard for some to see certain colours

~Allways do a spelchek

~ Beware of fancy backgrounds as these will distract

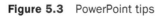

~ Use   to aid explanations

~ Only put bullet points on each slide, not lengthy explanations

~ Back up presentations with handouts

~ Keep it relatively short and put more information and references on handout

Figure 5.3   PowerPoint tips

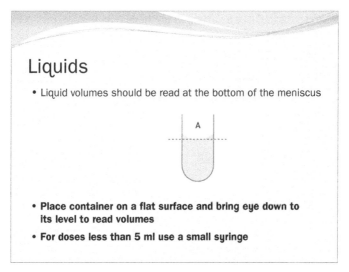

Figure 5.4   Example of a good PowerPoint slide

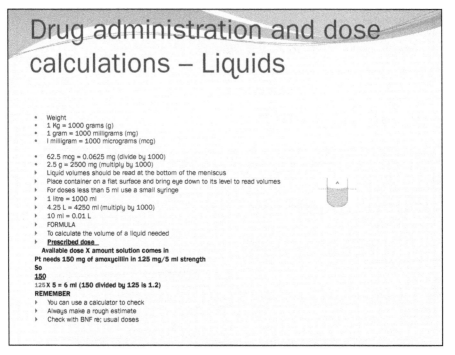

Figure 5.5   Example of a poor PowerPoint slide

- Key points are emphasised
- Presentation uses a variety of methods (e.g. lecture, group work, demonstration)
- Visual aids are used
- Presenter includes the audience and invites participation
- Presenter encourages questions and seeks group's experiences and opinions
- The learning is assessed
- The session is evaluated
- Presentation lasts no more than 40 minutes if no participation involved
- A handout is provided with references

Student's evaluation of a module

Awful. At times it was just so much information being thrown at you, no interaction just 'death by PowerPoint'.

Assessment of learning

We assess teaching sessions to determine how successful (or otherwise) they have been. We need to know if the learners have learnt! The method of assessment can depend upon what you have taught. By and large you can draw upon any of the methods suggested in Chapter 6 but for individual teaching sessions you will usually require a quickly applied measure of effectiveness at the end of each session, such as:

- Verbal question-and-answer session
- Short written question-and-answer test
- Multiple-choice test
- Discussion
- Practical test
- Observation of practice

Student evaluations

As well as assessing the students' knowledge from the session, we should assess the teaching style and methods used. Student evaluations are useful for checking that the session met its original aims and that the students benefited. This enables us to improve each time we do it. It also provides important feedback as to how we are developing as a teacher.

Student evaluation proforma

Student evaluation of teaching

- Were the aims and objectives clear?
- Were the aims and objectives met?
- Was the content understandable?
- Was the material linked to practice?
- Were the teaching methods appropriate?
- Did the session include student involvement and activity?
- Was the delivery interesting?
- Was the pace and timing alright?
- Was it well organised?

(continued)

- Were you invited to ask questions?

- Were the handouts useful?

- Any other comments/suggestions for improvement.

Questions teachers can ask themselves are:

- What went well?

- What didn't go well . . . how can I alter it for next time?

- Were the activities at the right level, too easy/too difficult?

- Was there sufficient student interaction and involvement?

- Were all involved?

Conclusion

There are a host of factors that go towards a successful teaching session. The following is a list of good practice advice, but if there were one thing we ought bear in mind, it is *variety*.

Summary of practical teaching tips

- Keep it simple (manageable chunks)

- Sequence it in a logical order

- Participation via group work tasks

- Demonstrate it

- Provide the opportunity for practice

- Make it fun

- Give praise

- Highlight the relevance to practice

- Summarise it and recap major points

- Evaluate it

- Reference it

- Give constructive feedback – what's done well and areas that need to developed

Summary

This chapter has:

- Shown how it is best to plan teaching according to specific aims and objectives

- Shown that there are a wide range of different teaching strategies at the mentor's disposal

- Suggested that variety is very important

- Identified that much good teaching is spontaneous and needs backing up with reflection

- Emphasised the need to evaluate our teaching

One of the best ways of measuring the effectiveness of teaching is by assessing the student's learning. The next chapter explores the ways in which we do this and looks at how we can do it in as fair and objective a way as possible.

References

Ausubel, D. (1978) *Educational Psychology: A cognitive view.* New York: Rinehart & Winston.

Bandura, A. (1977) *Social Learning Theory.* Englewood Cliffs, NJ: Prentice-Hall.

Biggs, J. (1999) *Teaching for Quality Learning at University.* Maidenhead: Society for Research into Education & Open University Press.

Bruner, J.S. (1966) *Towards a Theory of Instruction.* Cambridge, MA: Belknap Press.

Dewey, J. (1974) My pedagogic creed, in R. Archambault (ed.) *John Dewey on Education.* Chicago, IL: University of Chicago Press.

Dix, G. and Hughes, S. (2005) Teaching students in the classroom and clinical skills environment, *Nursing Standard,* 19(35): 41–7.

Eason, G., Stratford-Martin, J. and Atherton, H. (2012) An appraisal of the literature on teaching physical examination skills, *Education for Primary Care,* 23: 246–54.

Fry, H., Ketteridge, S. and Marshall, S. (eds.) (2003) *A Handbook for Teaching and Learning in Higher Education: Enhancing academic practice,* 2nd edn. London: Routledge Falmer.

Haidar, E. (2009) Clinical simulation: a better way of learning?, *Nursing Management*, 16(5): 22–3.

Larew, C., Lessans, S., Spunt, D., Foster, D. and Covington, B.G. (2006) Application of Benner's theory in an interactive patient care simulation, *Nursing Education Perspectives*, 27(1): 16–21.

Lewis, D.Y. and Ciak, A.D. (2011) The impact of a simulated lab experience for nursing students, *Nursing Education Perspectives*, 32(4): 256–8.

Ley, P. (1988) *Communicating with Patients: Improving communication, satisfaction and compliance*. London: Croom Helm.

Miller, G.A. (1956) The magical number seven, plus or minus two: some limits on our capacity for processing information, *Psychological Review*, 63(2): 81–97.

Nursing and Midwifery Council (NMC) (2008) *Standards to Support Learning and Assessment in Practice: NMC standards for mentors, practice teachers and teachers*, 2nd edn. London: NMC.

Oliver, R. and Endersby, C. (2000) *Teaching and Assessing Nurses: A handbook for preceptors*. London: Baillière Tindall.

Stables, I. (2012) Development of clinical skills: the contribution of peer learning, *Learning Disability Practice*, 15(8): 12–17.

Teasdale, K. (1993) Optimum use of limited resources: structured teaching in the clinical area, *Professional Nurse*, 9(3): 162–8.

6 Assessment: theory and practice reality

Key points

- Validity and reliability are the cornerstones of a fair and objective assessment
- Mentors need to be aware of the factors that can sway and influence an assessment
- Mentors need to ensure that their assessments are appropriate to the level the learner is at

NMC (2008) domains and outcomes for a mentor related to this chapter

Assessment and accountability

- Foster professional growth, personal development, and accountability through support of students in practice
- Demonstrate a breadth of understanding of assessment strategies and the ability to contribute to the total assessment process as part of the teaching team
- Provide constructive feedback to students and assist them in identifying future learning needs and actions
- Be accountable for confirming that students have met, or not met, the NMC competencies in practice

Evaluation of learning

- Contribute to evaluation of student learning and assessment experiences – proposing aspects for change as a result of such evaluation

Leadership

- Provide feedback about the effectiveness of learning and assessment in practice

Clinical assessment exercise

- Think about a student taking a pulse. What assessment criteria would you need to objectively assess that they were proficient?

- Draw up a list of criteria, including knowledge, skills, and attitudes. Suggest clear indicators that will demonstrate achievement of each criteria.

At the end of the chapter, check to see if your assessment meets the criteria discussed below.

This chapter examines the theory behind assessment and looks at how it can best be achieved in practice. Evidence suggests that assessment is often not the priority it ought to be. However, Hand (2006) states that assessment is crucial in protecting the public and maintaining the credibility of the profession, while Phillips et al. (2000) suggest that assessment is seen by many mentors as one of those activities that gets done only when the important tasks of the day, such as patient care, are completed.

First-year student on a mental health rehabilitation ward

I passed the placement but I had no real mentor, they all assumed I knew what I was doing. I had no initial or mid point interview and in the end the ward manager just signed my outcomes off. You couldn't really say that I was assessed.

Experienced mentor to novice mentor regarding a final placement student

I can't see how she got this far or understand why they didn't pick up on it in any of her previous placements – it must have been obvious. They obviously didn't assess her at all.

Theory of assessment

Definition of assessment

There is no completely adequate definition of assessment. Indeed, it is hard to try to define it because there are so many variables and variations, depending upon what or who you are trying to assess. The *Concise Oxford English Dictionary* states that to assess is to evaluate or estimate, while others suggest it is to judge or appraise the worth of something. These definitions are adequate because they embrace a wide range of situations and the reality is that we are indeed trying to make a judgement about the level of someone's ability. However, there are many other possibilities.

Variations on the theme

estimate	determine	measure	compare	score	value
appraise	grade	rate	ascertain	conclude	decide

While it is clear that we are trying to gauge the degree of learning, the focus of assessment can be upon many areas of learning, such as competence, knowledge, skills, attitudes, progress, performance, and so on. There are also different levels of achievement and competence, often defined by written standards and criteria that have to be met. In nursing, the assessment process is usually linked to the three areas of Bloom's taxonomy – knowledge, skills, and attitude.

In truth, the definition of assessment we use is also heavily dependent upon why we are assessing as well as what we are assessing. If I were to assess your level of competence at managing a shift, I would look at different criteria than if I were to assess your ability in mathematics compared with your peers. In the former, I would need to evaluate your management and communication skills, but also help you to decide where you are and what you need to do next. In the latter, I would need to score and measure your test results, to determine how you compare with your peers.

Purpose of assessment

Just as defining assessment is not straightforward, neither is the apparent purpose of assessment. Essentially, we assess in order to help people learn but in relation to a student nurse's clinical practice we assess for a variety of other reasons too:

- To monitor the student's progress
- To provide feedback
- To uncover learning needs
- To motivate the student
- To monitor their progress
- To assess their level of competence
- To assess knowledge, skills, and attitude
- To measure the effectiveness of our teaching
- To safeguard the patient and protect the public

Because we assess for a host of good reasons, the assessment process must be very robust. It needs to accurately enable us to make realistic judgements about the student's level of competence, and whether to pass them or not. For the student, a good assessment process also gives them valuable feedback. It helps them to identify where they are at, highlights deficits in their learning, identifies what they need to do, and enables them to set realistic future goals.

A good assessment process should also enable us to predict the future behaviour of the nurses we train. It should, if we pass them, enable us to be assured that they will perform successfully in a safe and professional manner using the latest evidence-based practice.

This is asking a lot of an assessment process, and no process is totally infallible. However, we can cut down the risks by ensuring that the assessment process itself meets certain standards and criteria that are considered best practice.

Cardinal criteria

There are several key elements to assessment that can improve its quality and render it more objective. These are called the 'cardinal criteria' and include validity, reliability, discrimination, practicality, and transparency.

Validity

The concept of validity asks several questions of an assessment and can be very difficult to demonstrate.

- Does the assessment measure what it's supposed to measure, i.e. the learning outcomes?

- Is the assessment appropriate to the level of the learner?

- Is what is being tested within the context of the course? Does it test what is actually in the curriculum? (Content validity)

- Does the assessment predict the future performance of the student? (Predictive validity)

- If two different assessments are used to assess the same thing, do they give the same result? If a student took both, would they get the same result? (Concurrent validity)

- Does the assessment reveal attitudes and values correctly? (Construct validity) The constructs of professionalism and attitude are important in nursing and during a placement there will be ample opportunity for the student to demonstrate these over a range of circumstances and in interactions with patients and other healthcare workers.

- Does the assessment appear to be relevant to what is being assessed? (Face validity) For example, assessing ability to perform aseptic technique via questions would not have face validity.

Question

How valid is assessing a student's ability to perform cardiopulmonary resuscitation by asking them to write an essay on it?

A test can, at times, merely assess the ability to undertake the test rather than the ability to practically apply knowledge. It can test the student's ability to memorise information rather than understand it.

Reliability

For an assessment to be valid, it must be also be reliable (i.e. consistent in its application). Reliability essentially means that an assessment gives similar results when repeated on different occasions. This is called *re-test reliability*.

If an assessment gives the same results when used by different assessors, it is also said to have *inter-rater reliability*.

Thus a good assessment should always give the same result no matter who is administering it and in different situations. Several things can hamper reliability, including biases on the part of the assessor, lack of time in practice to do the assessment fairly, the competence of the assessor, and others listed later.

Portfolios

The greater the variety and range of evidence within a portfolio, the more valid and reliable it will be. A range of opinion from others will also enhance the portfolio's validity and reliability as a form of assessment.

Length of placement

A common feature of mentor feedback is that some placements are too short to be able to make an adequate assessment of the student. Think about your own experiences, placements, and current clinical area in relation to this.

What strategies can be employed in short placements to make the assessments valid?

Discrimination

The assessment should clearly distinguish between those who are up to a certain standard and those who are not. It should distinguish between different levels of ability, between a good pass and a weak one. Put simply, it should tell us who can and who can't, who knows and who doesn't!

Practicality

The assessment should be practical to administer in terms of its ease of use, cost, and the time it takes. It should not be too difficult for teachers to administer and within the sphere of nursing this means it should take into account the needs of the busy clinical area and team.

Third-year student on acute medical unit

I felt that the management should have allocated time for the mentor to complete the final interview and discuss competencies. As it was very busy, there wasn't time during the shift to complete the documentation, therefore my mentor had to come to the ward during her annual leave to complete it.

Transparency

It should be clear to all learners exactly what the assessment is, they should be able to easily understand it, and the associated learning outcomes should be unambiguous. (See the discussion on subjectivity below.)

Types of assessment

It is possible to distinguish between different types of assessment, each of which has its own distinct purpose.

Continuous assessment

Oliver and Endersby (2000) suggest that no single final procedure is adequate for assessing clinical competence and so it is far better to assess continuously. Continuous assessment is assessment conducted over a period of time, rather than a single fixed test. Thus the student's day-to-day clinical practice is scrutinised for the duration of their placement, and not just tested in their last week. Good feedback should foster growth throughout the placement and the process of continuous assessment relies upon good working relationships between student and mentor. The feedback allows the student to monitor their progress towards achieving their learning objectives. It can be seen as subjective because of the bond that is formed between the mentor and student, which can lead perhaps to a more favourable appraisal than one made by an unknown assessor. It is also quite time-consuming for the mentor and a common feature of student placement evaluations is not having enough time with the mentor.

Continuous assessment consists of both formative and summative elements.

Formative assessment

Formative assessment occurs over a period of time and is used to help the student gain an idea of where they are and what they need to do to progress. It helps them to identify strengths and weaknesses and learning needs. The process is facilitated by the teacher or mentor providing regular feedback and praise, which also helps develop confidence and fosters motivation. The active involvement of the student in their learning is important here, as is self-assessment. The feedback fosters further learning by identifying gaps in knowledge and highlighting how these can be overcome. It also allows us to adjust the teaching to take into account any new learning needs. It can be useful to formalise the process at certain stages by jointly developing specific action plans.

Reflection is an essential aspect of formative assessment alongside questioning, discussion, and self-assessment. Such an approach is said to foster a deeper level of learning.

Summative assessment

Usually following a period of formative assessment, a summative assessment occurs at a fixed time and is used to determine if the student has reached the desired level or met the set criteria. It is ultimately the summative assessment that provides the employer, educational institution, and profession with evidence of competence. Because of this, the process of assessment must be rigorous, serving as it does to protect the public by ensuring that all who pass are of a certain standard.

Self-assessment

With self-assessment, the students set their own performance criteria and targets. It provides the learner with the opportunity to explore any gaps in their knowledge and identify both their learning needs and strategies to meet them. It is subjective in nature, but the views of others can be taken into account through discussion and questioning. Reflective practice is a key element of self-assessment. Mentors should thus provide regular opportunities for students to reflect upon activities and clinical situations they have experienced. Such reflective discussions do not always have to be formalised or long. In the community, they often take place on the journey between visits, but occasionally the need will arise for a more formalised and undisturbed examination of a scenario between mentor and student. Such a discussion can then be written up and related to the literature and presented as evidence in the student's portfolio. Discussion in relation to reflection and frameworks for reflection can be found in Chapter 7, 'Building a portfolio of evidence'. Having identified new learning needs via reflection and self-assessment, action plans are a good way of translating these insights into practical instructions necessary to achieve that learning.

Two useful aids to self-assessment are a self-penned action plan and a more detailed SWOT analysis.

Example of an action plan

Action plan

- What area do I need to improve upon?
- What do I need to achieve specifically in relation to knowledge, skills, and attitude?
- How will I achieve this?
- What resources and help do I need?
- Target date

Action plans can of course be much more detailed with the broad goals broken down so that each specific sub-goal has its own action plan. For a discussion of the value of learning contracts, see Chapter 5, 'Teaching in practice'.

Reflective action plan

A reflective action plan can be used to analyse a clinical experience the student has had.

Reflective action plan

- What went well?
- What didn't?
- What learning needs have I identified?
- How will I meet them?

SWOT analysis

This has been discussed in detail in Chapters 2 and 3 in relation to the mentor's own skills and the learning environment. It is a good idea here for mentors to encourage a student to carry out a SWOT analysis of their learning needs in relation to a placement. This can then be used to form the basis of an action plan. The following is an example of a SWOT analysis.

Learning and competence

- What STRENGTHS do I bring to this placement?

- What WEAKNESSES can I perceive in my ability and knowledge?

- What OPPORTUNITIES can I use to aid my learning and overcome these?

- What THREATS might get in the way and how can I overcome them?

Second-year student on surgical ward

I was grateful to my mentor because I had real problems early on and didn't say anything. She saw it and took me aside and did an action plan with me that made me focus on important areas. In the end I passed, but without a good mentor I would have just carried on and failed.

Criterion-referenced assessment

A criterion-referenced assessment is used to assess a student against predetermined criteria, such as the NMC competencies. These provide standards against which we can judge students.

Such an assessment avoids many of the pitfalls of subjectivity, such as the 'halo and horn effect' (see below). With criterion-referenced assessment, the student should be clear as to what they need to do.

Norm-referenced assessment

Norm-referenced assessment is used to compare one person with another or with a group of peers at the same level, or with an expected level of attainment for a similar group of learners. Such an assessment is open to the biases of the 'halo and horn effect' (see below). The focus can veer away from the specific outcomes and fall upon the student's comparability with fellow students.

Peer assessment

Just as teaching your peers can be a great learning experience, being assessed by your peers can be a great motivator. It is particularly useful in enabling students to gain formative feedback relating to their performance in practice. Most mentor training courses link the budding mentor with a qualified mentor who is charged with assessing that they have met the NMC domains for mentors. Similarly, many buddy schemes have junior nursing students mentored by more senior students. This can provide a less threatening experience than performing under the eye of the mentor and for some students this will be a welcome opportunity. Having students of the same level assess each other is also a very useful way of helping them to become more familiar with the assessment criteria and assess their own level of knowledge. One other benefit of peer assessment is that it can make students think more deeply about how to provide constructive feedback.

Evaluating learning

This topic was covered in Chapter 5, 'Teaching in practice', but it is worth trying to apply the cardinal criteria of assessment to teaching session evaluations.

Assessing your teaching

Think of a teaching session you do with students or an experience you provide them with and devise an assessment tool to provide you with feedback as to how much they have learnt.

Next, consider if the tool is valid, reliable, practical, and discriminating!

Factors influencing assessments

There are many ways in which an assessment can be influenced for good or for bad. An understanding of these factors can help to keep the assessment as fair and objective as possible.

What gets in the way?

Try and identify factors that might influence or invalidate an assessment of a student in a clinical setting.

How might these be overcome?

Halo effect

A halo effect occurs when favourable prior knowledge of a student leads the assessor to make a more favourable judgement. Something that a student excelled in in a previous placement area might lead a mentor to assume competence and not test it thoroughly once more.

Horn effect

The horn effect is the opposite of the halo effect, where prior knowledge of an unfavourable kind leads the mentor to make a more negative judgement.

Hawthorne effect

The Hawthorne effect is a sociological phenomenon named after the factory in which the workers were being studied. This effect reflects that we tend to perform better when we are being observed or are being given special attention.

Error of leniency

This is simply being too lenient or soft and tending to ignore or overlook mistakes. It is giving people the benefit of the doubt.

Error of severity

This is the opposite of the error of leniency – being too harsh, overly critical, and picking up on minor errors.

Central tendency error

This means awarding middle grades irrespective of the quality of the work or performance. This can be seen as 'playing it safe' and not being willing to give extremely high or low scores. This is often a criticism levelled at the marking of academic assignments.

Discussion: subjectivity

It is difficult to come up with an assessment process that has clear and specific criteria and yet is also adaptable to many different clinical environments.

(continued)

Frith and Macintosh (1984) suggest a good assessment rids us of the influence of the assessor as a person, thus raising the assessment's reliability.

There is an element of subjectivity in most assessment procedures. The NMC competencies, for example, are often quite vague and can be said to be open to wide interpretation. This is a little worrying from a public protection point of view. Different mentors might have different expectations and interpretations of what is expected. Many placement areas have mapped the outcomes to specific learning experiences to reduce the risk of misinterpretation and to ease the understanding of the competency wording. In one respect, it is beneficial to have vague criteria because it enables them to be adapted and applied to many different settings. On the other hand, strictly defined criteria are easier to understand and make decisions about.

You will probably remember being surprised that a fellow student passed a placement, or that a fellow mentor passed a student who you thought should have failed. Maybe it was an error of leniency or central tendency, or maybe it was because the outcomes were too vague so that it would have been unfair to fail someone.

What do you think? Should the competencies be vague or sharply defined? Should they be open to interpretation or should we be using a strict checklist? Look carefully at the field competencies and see if you fully understand what is being asked of each one.

Subjectivity and bias: can you be a mentor to everyone?

We are supposed to be professionals and able to work with a wide variety of different people and other staff. But we are also fallible and human.

Honesty is important in nursing and assessment, and occasionally there may be a 'clash of personalities' that renders the mentoring difficult and assessment unfair. Even the most objective person knows someone who they cannot relate to or work with for whatever reason. If you sense this is the case, you should arrange for another mentor to take over in the interests of fairness and objectivity. It's a two-way street and occasionally there will be a student who finds you difficult to work with. This should be openly discussed and if it can't be resolved the student should be handed over to another mentor.

Assessment in practice

There are many different methods of assessment that mentors can use in practice to assess the clinical competence of their students.

Observation of practical skills

The mentor's direct observation of the student's practice is the cornerstone of nursing assessment, mirroring a long tradition of vocational training whereby the master craftsman carefully observes the progress of the
apprentice. It is strong evidence of competence because the mentor can see
for themselves what the student can or can't do rather than relying upon the
word of others or indirect evidence such as a discussion. Alongside practical skills, observation will also highlight attitudes and ability to respond
to different situations and adapt practice to individual circumstances using
decision-making and problem-solving skills. Over the duration of a placement, many opportunities will arise for such skills and their application to
be observed in a variety of settings and circumstances, thus increasing the
predictive validity of such an assessment.

> *Most assessment of competence should be undertaken through direct
> observation in practice (Standards to Support Learning and Assess-
> ment in Practice, NMC 2008).*

Questioning

Questioning occurs in a variety of circumstances. Mentors ask students
questions during shared procedures and throughout the day-to-day routine,
helping to give the mentor an indication of the student's level of knowledge
and understanding. Questioning can also be formalised and carried out as
an assessment, either formative or summative. Another variation is a set of
printed questions the student takes away, thinks about, and responds to,
which can form the basis of a discussion at a later date. If observation is the
cornerstone of assessing practical skills, then questioning is the lynchpin of
assessing the student's knowledge base.

> I keep six honest serving men
> (They taught me all I knew);
> Their names are What and Why and When
> And How and Where and Who.
>
> Rudyard Kipling

The words who, what, why, where, when, and how are good ones to bear in
mind when framing questions. For a brief discussion of useful types of questions, refer back to Chapter 2, 'The effective mentor'.

Bloom

Bloom's (1956) taxonomy is useful here, too, as it breaks the cognitive domain down into six levels of understanding, and questions can be pitched at these levels to match the level the student is at and also to challenge them to think more deeply about the subject.

- Knowledge (recalling information and facts)
  List, define, describe, arrange, label
  List the major types of dementia

- Comprehension (understanding meaning, interpreting)
  Explain, summarise, discuss, critique
  Explain the difference between Alzheimer's disease and multi-infarct dementia

- Application (putting into practice)
  Apply, solve, construct, manage
  How can reality orientation help Jim to maintain his independence?

- Analysis (examining something's structure, elements and their interrelationships)
  Compare, relate, break down, contrast
  What are the relative advantages and disadvantages of reality orientation compared with validation approaches to dementia?

- Synthesis (using it and creating your own variation or adaptation)
  Plan, propose, design, revise
  Devise a plan of care for Jim giving a rationale for the approach adopted

- Evaluation (measuring effectiveness)
  Review, assess, appraise, justify
  Evaluate the effectiveness of Jim's care plan

Reflective discussion/writing

Much of what needs to be explored in relation to reflection is covered in Chapter 7, 'Building a portfolio of evidence'. Here, we briefly examine its important role as evidence of competence. Students will vary widely in their opinion as to the value of reflection and their ability to undertake it; often reflection will need to be encouraged by the mentor. There is also an assumption that learning occurs after reflection, but this is only the case if the mentor helps the student to probe and explore the issues in depth. As with testimonies (see below), the student should accompany reflective writing and notes from reflective discussions with a short explanation of how it relates to and meets their competencies. Reflective sessions and writing are often formative but can also be summative when presented as evidence of achievement. They can indicate self-awareness, knowledge, attitude, and ability to apply theory to practice.

Case studies and case presentations/care plan reviews

These are an excellent way of gauging the student's integration of theory with practice and of assessing and enhancing their communication skills. Working alone or in pairs, students should be encouraged to undertake an in-depth study of a client of particular interest to them. This reappraisal of the client and the care they are receiving should then be presented to the team or a small group. Presentation and teaching skills are thus also incorporated into such a task, but it is the student's ability to link theory with practice and appraise care that is the most important aspect of this assessment. A variation on this theme, instead of reviewing the full case history and care of a client, is to ask the student to review the care plan, reassess the client or check the assessments and review the goals and outcomes, and rewrite the care plan. The student should then present this and engage the team in debate with the support of their mentor.

Group work

The ability to work as part of a team is crucial in modern health care and there are many group tasks students can be asked to undertake when there are several students on the same placement. One that will be of particular value to the mentor, and team, is to ask the students to review the student information pack, or learning objectives for the area. Other tasks could be to review new policies, procedures, equipment, drugs, and therapy, or examine the evidence base for practice. Such tasks can then also be presented as above and students can use these as evidence for their own portfolios.

Presentations

These are another variation on the above two themes. The student will likely have come across many things in the classroom which are new to the ward staff, or will have had experiences on placement elsewhere which they can share with the team by way of an update, teaching session or discussion. Often work they have prepared for class-based presentations can be presented to the team.

Student self-assessment

This is described above and mentors should encourage students to perform self-assessments as the basis for discussion with the mentor in relation to identifying their learning needs and goals for the placement.

Learning contracts

Learning contracts are very useful following on from student self-assessments and are discussed in Chapter 5, 'Teaching in practice'.

Testimony of others

The opinions of fellow professionals and others will serve to make any assessment fairer and more objective. The wider the source of opinion and range of evidence the better. This is especially so when the scenario is one of a failing student. The views of associate mentors, colleagues, members of the multidisciplinary team, clients, carers, healthcare assistants, and others can all be drawn upon. The student can be encouraged to solicit statements regarding their own performance from others they have worked with or on insight visits they have undertaken. This can represent a sound body of evidence when the student writes a short accompanying passage explaining how the testimony relates to their competencies. A wider body of opinion will increase both the validity and reliability of the evidence.

Portfolios

These are discussed in detail in Chapter 7, 'Building a portfolio of evidence'. The purpose and structure of portfolios are discussed alongside an examination of the nature of the evidence a student can provide. However, it is important to reiterate here that it is the student's responsibility to demonstrate their competence to the mentor and convince them they have achieved their outcomes by taking them through and explaining their portfolio evidence.

Essential skills clusters

Following consultation related to fitness for practice issues, the NMC introduced the idea of essential skills clusters (NMC 2007). The consultation had suggested that recently qualified nurses lacked confidence and competence in certain key skills. The essential skills clusters (ESCs) are generic statements of skills outcomes required to enter the field and competencies required to enter the register. The ESCs complement the existing NMC competencies and can be said to reflect the skills the public expect newly qualified nurses to have. They became compulsory elements of the pre-registration nursing curriculum in 2008 and were amended in the *Standards for Pre-registration Nursing Education* in 2010.

The ESCs cover skills in the key areas of:

- care, compassion, and communication
- organisational aspects of care
- infection prevention and control
- nutrition and fluid management
- medicine management

(continued)

The clusters focus upon baseline assessments and calculations in these areas.

These skills are linked to progression points at the end of the first and second years and for entry to the register. They support the competencies and can be mapped against specific competencies in the domains. Education providers decide which skills to assess in practice or by simulation, and the number of attempts a student is allowed. Annex 3 of the new pre-registration standards (NMC 2010) includes specific indicators that can be used to develop checklists by education providers. This is akin to a second set of competencies and although it somewhat complicates the paperwork, it should ensure greater safety and overall competence in the newly qualified nurse.

Mentors should become familiar with the education provider's guidelines, which should identify the specific criteria the student needs to achieve in order to pass each skill at each progression point. It is also wise to identify early on in a placement which skills assessments a student needs to undertake while with you. This will allow you to ensure that sufficient practices can be arranged and dates for summative assessments can be fixed well in advance.

Levels of learner and competencies

The NMC (2004) defined competence as having the skills and ability to practise safely and effectively without the need for constant supervision. This was refined in 2010 as follows: 'the combination of skills, knowledge and attitudes, values and technical abilities that underpin safe and effective nursing practice and interventions' (NMC 2010, p. 145)

There are four sets of NMC competencies:

- Professional values
- Communication and interpersonal skills
- Nursing practice and decision-making
- Leadership, management, and decision-making

Each of these sets of competencies comprises generic and field-specific competencies.

The NMC competencies are designed to take the student through levels of ability from non-nurse to proficient. Certain criteria have to be met to move from the first year into the fields and then further criteria have to be met to gain registration.

Most nurse training courses elaborate upon this by identifying further levels, sometimes per semester and sometimes per year. Several models and taxonomies of levels of competency and participation are used nationally. One such model commonly used is that of Bondy (1983), who examined rating scales in clinical education in relation to competencies and many nurse education courses have adopted and adapted his work. Nurse education courses identify the levels at which students must demonstrate achievement of competence in relation to knowledge, skills, and attitudes.

Bondy identified five levels of competency: dependent, marginal, assisted, supervised, and independent. These have been modified by nursing courses to a simpler format such as that below.

Level 1 (start of first year)
Practises with constant supervision

Level 2 (end of CFP)
Practises with assistance

Level 3 (end of year 2)
Practises with decreasing supervision, requiring occasional support and prompts

Level 4 (before progression to registration)
Practises independently, meeting the standards of competence, seeking advice and support as appropriate

At each of these levels within the four sets there are usually a series of more well-defined indicators of what constitutes adequate performance in order to help mentors make decisions about the student's competence. For example, at Level 1 the student will be developing communication skills but at Level 4 they are expected to communicate effectively with the nursing team and other professionals.

Attitude

The academic side of nursing is mostly assessed in the university while clinical 'hands-on' skills are tested thoroughly on placement. Alongside these clinical skills, professional behaviour, teamwork, caring, attitude, and motivation should also be assessed. However, it is the attitude aspect of nursing that tends to suffer most from poor assessment or falling under the radar. Errors of leniency seem to come into play here and evidence suggests that we do not place as much emphasis upon this aspect as we do the knowledge and skills aspects of nursing. We should be assessing the student's compassion, respect, caring, honesty, integrity, reliability, and enthusiasm, but often overlook these.

Reflective piece by a nurse on mentorship course

We recently had a student who wasn't meeting the standards. Their clinical skills were satisfactory but their whole attitude towards nursing was questionable at times. She lacked motivation and had little enthusiasm to further her knowledge base. It left me with a dilemma, as there was nothing specific that I could have failed them on, it was difficult to quantify exactly what the problem was.

And another . . .

There was an awkward student who was never coming in on time and didn't seem to care at all. They were rude to patients and treated the nursing assistants like they were worthless. It was all in their attitude. Their mentor didn't know how best to approach the student without getting personal. In the end she got the link tutor involved and they arranged a meeting between all three of them and helped the mentor point things out. The student didn't change much but the link tutor came back for the final interview and that made it much easier for the mentor, otherwise I think they would have passed.

The question of 'attitude' is an important one and it is an area we will discuss in detail in Chapter 8, 'Supporting failing students'.

Who can assess?

The NMC are clear in relation to who can assess nursing and midwifery students. Registrants from any profession can be involved in formative assessment. Indeed, it is good practice to gather as wide a range of opinion as possible by utilising colleagues, other professionals, healthcare assistants, and so on. It was noted in Chapter 1 that the modern nurse interacts routinely with a wide range of other healthcare professionals, and the 2010 NMC *Standards for Preregistration Nursing Education* embrace this fact. At progression points 1 and 2, assessment can be by a nurse in any field. At progression point 3, entry to the register, the assessor must be a 'sign-off mentor' nurse on the same part of the register the student is wishing to enter. However, other registered healthcare professionals who have been suitably prepared can supervise and contribute towards the assessment of nursing students (see Chapter 1).

Levels and evidence-based practice

What often lets students down is their evidence base. They can have good practical skills but find it hard to justify their use and often find it hard to adapt them from one setting to another, such as hospital to community. A student can be asked the simple question 'why do we do this?', and be tasked with providing the evidence. This is a useful two-way process, as it involves not only the identification of the evidence but a discussion as to its robustness and its usefulness. The blind application of evidence is not always prudent, as the setting and client may differ and so the approach must be adapted.

Ongoing achievement record

The ongoing achievement record (OAR) is the local education centre/ university version of the student's documentation indicating achievement of competencies over the whole three years. This is to enable the sign-off mentor to have an overview of the student's total training. The OAR will accompany the student from placement to placement and thus be available for each mentor to see. Education providers are bound to obtain the student's consent that this will be shared between mentors. The downside of this is students having a 'bad' placement through no fault of their own – a personality clash, for example, leading to an unfavourable report. This negative report would then be seen by all future mentors, which could be deemed unfair and the 'horn' effect might be invoked. However, we must assume that mentors are objective professionals and will not make negative pre-judgements, but form their own opinion of the student. The main reason for sharing of past performance is that it allows the mentor to identify any areas of concern from previous placements or knowledge and skill deficits that need to be addressed.

Besides having pages with previous competencies signed off, the OAR will also contain comments upon the student's overall performance, enthusiasm, and professionalism. It is the student's responsibility to ensure that this document is completed and it should be used by the student and mentor to set goals and an action plan at the beginning of a placement.

Good practice in assessment

Although it could be argued that it is the student's responsibility for identifying their own learning needs and self-assessment, the mentor needs to ensure that certain aspects of the assessment process are adhered to in order to provide a fair and objective assessment.

Good practice guidelines for assessment

- Ensure that you assess all three domains – knowledge, skills, *and* attitude.
- Observe your learner.

(continued)

- Use associate mentors, and seek the opinions of colleagues so that the assessment is not just yours, but that of the team. Arrange for the student to have insight visits and to work with other healthcare and associated staff.

- Listen to the student.

- At the initial interview, ensure you understand the student's learning outcomes and that they understand your expectations and the assessment plan, and what you will be looking for as evidence of achievement.

- Set dates for intermediate and final interviews so that the student is aware of these well in advance and thus can prepare themselves adequately.

- Identify placement-specific outcomes and the student's individual learning goals.

- Identify which 'essential skills' the student must achieve and set dates for the summative assessment.

- Encourage students to self-assess.

- Ensure you work with the student for a sufficient amount of time.

- Meet with them regularly to review their evidence and achievement instead of leaving it all to the final interview.

- Ensure you broker sufficient learning experiences.

- Provide constructive feedback frequently and as soon as possible after an event.

- Ask them questions such as Kipling's who, what, why, when, where, and how!

- Ask them what they think about their experiences in frequent reflective discussions.

- Ask them to analyse their own performance.

- Concentrate on the positives.

- Help to overcome any negatives.

- At the mid-point interview, identify strengths and progress and areas in need of attention/problem areas. As well as knowledge and skills, pay due regard to professionalism, attitude, timekeeping, and interpersonal skills. Confirm the date of the final interview.

- Liaise with higher education staff if there are significant concerns about performance.

- Put in place an action plan with clear goals to overcome any deficiencies.

- Provide the opportunity for deficiencies to be overcome.

- Provide support and reassurance.

Do I need a degree to assess a student on a degree programme?

No, the NMC only requires that the mentor hold a *professional* qualification equal to or higher than the level the student is working towards. More importantly, however, is the ability of the mentor to demonstrate that they are underpinning their practice with up-to-date evidence. Being able to undertake a literature search is an important aspect of this. Nurses should come across as problem-solvers, searching for possible solutions and trying them out and adapting them to their own circumstances and clients. Taking this a step further will see them publishing their findings and variations and so adding to the body of knowledge. Mentors play an important role here in fostering this enquiring ethos in students and showing them how to access relevant databases. Thus although you don't necessarily need a degree, you do need some good academic skills such as literature searching and the ability to appraise the evidence that literature throws up. The ability to conduct a literature search and appraise the evidence will be examined in Chapter 10.

Summary

This chapter has:

- Looked at the cardinal criteria for an objective assessment

- Looked at how assessment can be skewed

- Looked at the most common types of assessment

- Summarised good practice in assessment

Having looked at assessment and the various forms it can take, it is now time to examine the presentation of that evidence. Chapter 7 looks at the concept of the portfolio from the perspective of both the student and mentor.

Further reading

Hand, H. (2006) Assessment of learning in clinical practice, *Nursing Standard*, 21(4): 48–56. An excellent article summarising best practice in assessment and the underlying principles.

Rowntree, D. (1997) *Assessing Students: How shall we know them?* London: Kogan Page. This is a classic text on assessment that is full of insight and wisdom.

West, S., Clark, T. and Jasper, M. (eds.) (2007) *Enabling Learning in Nursing and Midwifery Practice*. Chichester: Wiley. This book contains an excellent chapter on assessment of practice, which clearly explains the principles and frames them in the practice context.

References

Bloom, B.S. (1956) *Taxonomy of Educational Objectives, Handbook I: The cognitive domain.* New York: David McKay.

Bondy, N.K. (1983) Criterion-referenced definitions for rating scales in clinical education, *Journal of Nursing Education,* 22(9): 376–82.

Frith, D. and Macintosh, H.G. (1984) *A Teacher's Guide to Assessment.* Cheltenham: Stanley Thornes.

Hand, H. (2006) Assessment of learning in clinical practice, *Nursing Standard,* 21(4): 48–56.

Nursing and Midwifery Council (NMC) (2004) *Standards of Proficiency for Pre-registration Nursing Education.* London: NMC.

Nursing and Midwifery Council (NMC) (2007) *Essential Skills Clusters for Pre-registration Nursing Programmes.* NMC Circular 07/2007. Annexe 1 and Annexe 2. London: NMC.

Nursing and Midwifery Council (NMC) (2008) *Standards to Support Learning and Assessment in Practice: NMC standards for mentors, practice teachers and teachers,* 2nd edn. London: NMC.

Nursing and Midwifery Council (NMC) (2010) *Standards for Pre-registration Nursing Education.* London: NMC. Available at: http://standards.nmc-uk.org/PublishedDocuments/Standards%20for%20pre-registration%20nursing%20education%2016082010.pdf [accessed 2 March 2014].

Oliver, R. and Endersby, C. (2000) *Teaching and Assessing Nurses: A handbook for preceptors.* London: Baillière Tindall.

Phillips, T., Schostak, J., Tyler, J. and Allen, L. (2000) *Practice and Assessment: An evaluation of the assessment of practice at diploma, degree and postgraduate level in pre- and post-registration nursing and midwifery education.* London: English National Board.

7 Building a portfolio of evidence

NMC (2008b) domains and outcomes for a mentor related to this chapter

Assessment and accountability

- Foster professional growth, personal development, and accountability through support of students in practice

Evaluation of learning

- Participate in self and peer evaluation to facilitate personal development, and contribute to the development of others

This chapter identifies a range of evidence that both budding mentors and student nurses can use to demonstrate achievement of their competencies. Having to develop their own portfolio allows the budding mentor to appreciate the process their students will be going through. Most pre-registration nursing courses encourage students to compile portfolios and use them as a form of assessment of practice competencies. Many of the exercises and activities here can be adapted for mentors to use with their students, thus helping students to achieve their competencies.

What is a portfolio?

A basic definition is that a portfolio is a collection of evidence of experiences and learning a person has undertaken.

> *A set of pieces of creative work intended to demonstrate a person's ability (Compact Oxford English Dictionary 2005).*

Beyond registration, nurses keep a portfolio as a record of their continuing professional development. This is a mandatory requirement of registration in the UK. Post-registration education and practice (PREP) are standards of continued professional development set by the NMC (2008a). Currently, this is set at a minimum of five days or 35 hours over three years. The qualified nurse's portfolio should demonstrate the achievement of this.

The PREP Handbook (NMC 2008a)

Visit this online at www.nmc-uk.org and read through it. It contains useful material relating to what learning activities can be undertaken in different clinical environments and evidence of their relevance.

Portfolios are usually compiled when engaged in work-based learning, as in nurse education, but they can be personal documents relating to any or all aspects of an individual's life, personal or professional.

In relation to nursing, McMullen and colleagues' (2003, p. 288) definition comes closest to describing a portfolio: 'A collection of evidence, usually in written form, of both the products and processes of learning. It attests to achievements and personal and professional development, by providing critical analysis of its content.'

Educationally, the collection of evidence is usually backed up with critical reflection upon experiences had and learning undertaken. This reflection helps the student to identify key aspects of the learning and areas worthy of exploration. It is quite a task to compile a good portfolio and the compilation of one is seen as an important, educationally robust learning method. A poor student will place a selection of semi-relevant articles and photocopied material into a file and present it as evidence of learning, but without a critical and reflective analysis the collection will be virtually worthless from an educational point of view.

Many nursing students are daunted by the thought of having to compile a portfolio, because as Timmins (2008) suggests, they are somewhat used to being spoon-fed via lectures and the portfolio is often their first experience of self-directed learning. Timmins asks her readers to think about how much they were involved in their last lecture and what they learnt, and to contrast this with a project they had to complete on their own. The reality is usually that the project involved them more and made them learn more, and this is part of the rationale behind a portfolio.

Basic features and aims of a portfolio

- **Personal:** It is a personal document, uniquely relating to your own experiences and learning. You compile it as you see fit and in a style which suits you. There are no standard formats, only guidelines. It can be both professional and personal, related to many aspects of your life or just one.

- **Self-directed:** Essentially, the portfolio is under the compiler's direction, but we all need guidance and this is a key aspect of the role of the mentor. A good mentor can help a student to reflect and explore and thus identify learning needs.

- **Learning:** The portfolio is essentially a learning tool, it helps you to examine the experiences you have had, reflect upon them, apply knowledge to practice, identify your new learning needs, and demonstrate this progress to others if necessary.

- **Critical reflection:** It uses critical reflection as a learning tool. Boud et al. (1985) see reflection as the key to 'learning from experience', specifically in the working environment. Many educational theories relate to reflection, including that of Kolb (1984) discussed in Chapter 4. Put simply, you have an experience, reflect upon it and form a new opinion, try it out and reflect upon the new results and so on in a cyclical fashion (see section on 'Reflection' below). The fact that a portfolio forces you to learn to reflect is one of its key benefits.

- **Self-awareness:** The process of building a portfolio and its necessary reflective elements can only serve to heighten self-awareness and the responsibility for one's own needs and learning.

- **Learning needs:** It helps students to identify their own learning needs. These needs arise out of the critical reflection upon their experiences and practice. How can I progress, what do I need to learn next, how can I build upon this? Such reflection allows us to identify future learning objectives. This realisation allows us to identify specific learning experiences we need. The portfolio should also identify the student's strengths.

- **Developing critical skills:** A portfolio and the reflection undertaken help a student to explore the links between theory and practice. The portfolio process helps students review their existing knowledge as well as challenge assumptions they might hold. The dual nature of nurse education, 50% theory and 50% practice, means that the reflection undertaken in portfolio work is an important way of examining the links between the two, and exploring the relevance of the theory to the reality of practice. In this way, reflection helps to develop critical thinking and analytical, problem-solving skills.

(continued)

- **Outcomes:** The portfolio should demonstrate the achievement of competencies. Each entry should be cross-referenced to the outcomes it relates to.

- **Career enhancement:** The portfolio is a useful document to present at interview to back up your application. It is also a useful document to use when having an appraisal, as it should contain evidence of your ongoing achievements.

Structure of a portfolio

The NMC (2004) suggested that nursing students build a portfolio as part of their training. The NMC (2010) *Standards for Pre-registration Nursing Education* state that nurses must 'keep their knowledge and skills up to date through continuing professional development' but do not specifically require the development of a portfolio. However, a portfolio is very much the norm and each School of Nursing will have its own guidelines for portfolio compilation and structure. There is no nationally preferred format.

Exercise

Contact your educational representative or link tutor and find out what the local guidance is and what your students are being taught.

The structure of a portfolio is a matter of personal choice, but most student portfolios include certain key components. The structure can be modified beyond registration to replace some of the nurse training aspects with continuing professional development material. For nurse education purposes, it has been suggested that the portfolio be divided into sections according to the NMC domains of competency: Professional values, Communication and interpersonal skills, Nursing practice and decision making, and Leadership, management and team working. Some nursing students structure according to semesters, others use a simple academic and placement split.

Whatever the structure, the portfolio should be kept in a robust file, a large ring binder being excellent for this purpose. Other useful tips are that it should be separated into defined sections using dividers and that plastic pockets are useful for putting leaflets in and protecting articles.

The budding mentor's portfolio will obviously be geared to the mentor standards and can be structured in that way with a section for each standard. An alternative approach is to divide the portfolio according to the type of evidence, each piece of evidence being cross-referenced to the standards they refer to. This is the preferred option, as many pieces of evidence will refer to a number of the standards and their sub-clauses.

Sections within a portfolio

The list below includes sections that relate to a student's portfolio and a registered nurse's portfolio. Mentors compiling a portfolio might want to include some of these, but a general rule is that you need only include that which is relevant to the learning outcomes intended to be met by the portfolio. Remember that any evidence such as an article or a leaflet needs to be accompanied by a short explanation as to how it demonstrates achievement of the learning outcomes.

- Title page
- Index
- Curriculum vitae (including education and work history)
- Personal and professional goals
- Certificates (photocopies)
- Personal achievements outside of nursing (e.g. hobbies, sport, voluntary work)
- Course work
- Academic record/grade profile
- Case studies
- Essays or feedback sheets
- Reflective writing
- Critical incident analysis
- Question and answer
- Articles
- Leaflets
- Direct observations by mentors
- Insight visits
- SWOT analysis
- Testimonials or witness statements, i.e. the opinion of others
- Placement records/competency documents
- Policies, standards, protocols, etc.
- Courses, seminars, conferences attended
- Publications

e-portfolios

Increasing use is being made of portfolios kept on electronic devices and many software packages are available offering a variety of ways of managing and presenting a portfolio. Just like paper portfolios, they provide a vehicle for learning. However, e-portfolios are capable of many extra features and are less cumbersome. They can link to web sites and articles, and enable you to incorporate downloaded graphics, photographs, and other e-learning tools. They have the advantage of allowing for increasingly personalised ways of working and building and structuring the portfolio. In this way, they are dynamic and easy to update. They present new ways of viewing information and of presenting evidence to others. A bonus is their capacity to incorporate and link to discussions and interest groups. This networking promotes sharing of ideas and views, which in turn increases the possibilities for reflection by one's self and with others. An e-portfolio can support work-based learning through remote access to mentors, teachers, and others who can send information, tasks, prompts, and comments to areas they are allowed access to. It can be a useful way to showcase and profile your professional development, achievements, and career to date, as well as developing personal development and action plans. Nurses have a professional requirement to maintain a portfolio of evidence to show that they are updating their knowledge and skills. The NMC PREP (Post-registration education and practice) (NMC 2011) requirements are intended to help nurses maintain a high standard of practice, keep up to date with new developments, reflect and demonstrate that they are developing their practice. Because the pace of change is fast these days, an e-portfolio offers the best method of keeping pace with these changes. Constantly updating a hard copy portfolio can be quite time-consuming and after a while it will become very bulky. The use of an iPad, laptop or similar device will make the process much easier. Because such devices can store large quantities of information, they also help maintain an evidence-based practice approach with nurses being able to store relevant evidence in the form of papers and articles, NICE guidelines, etc., and update them as and when fresh evidence arises. Student nurses will be impressed by a mentor who is able to bring up a databank of research papers on an iPad!

There are many good web-based resources related to e-portfolios (see www.nhseportfolios.org) and it is only a matter of time before universities abandon paper portfolios altogether in favour of electronic ones for nurse education.

See Dion and Smolenski's (2008) article, 'Why you need an electronic professional portfolio', at http://www.americannursetoday.com/article.aspx?id=5598&fid=5558. They present a persuasive argument as to why we need to adopt the electronic approach.

Reflection

> The *Compact Oxford English Dictionary* (2005) defines reflection as 'serious thought or consideration'.

There is an unashamed emphasis upon reflection in current nursing literature. Reflective diaries, reflective discussions, and reflective writing appear to be the key to a meaningful education. Evidence from such reflective writing and discussions are a key element of much portfolio work. So we must answer the questions, what is reflection and why is it important? We also need to look at how it can best be achieved in practice given that one of the hardest aspects of mentoring students is finding the time for reflection and discussion. A discussion in the car following a community visit is a golden opportunity, and students should be mindful of the need to write up such discussions as evidence.

Reflection involves describing an event or experience in some detail, and analysing and evaluating one's thoughts, actions, and beliefs. The related theory can be examined in the light of this experience and new understanding. This is why nurses and nurse educators value reflection; as Fitzgerald and Chapman (2000) say, 'the approach focuses upon practice and values experience'.

Most people find it easier to use a model of reflection, of which there are many. However, despite the many models of reflection, it remains a personal learning style and the literature can offer only guidance. Learning in this way can be a rather slow process, as events and theory are mulled over in an attempt to make sense of something new. Kolb's (1984) experiential learning cycle suggests that reflection is an essential aspect of learning (see Figure 7.1). According to Kolb, learning from experience involves four stages in a cycle:

1. The student reflects on an experience, and then examines how they felt about it and how it went.

2. They then think about it, trying to understand it better by looking at the theory and why it happened that way.

3. They start to form new ideas about how it might be done differently so as to achieve a better outcome.

4. They then try out these new ideas and experiment with variations arising from their reflection.

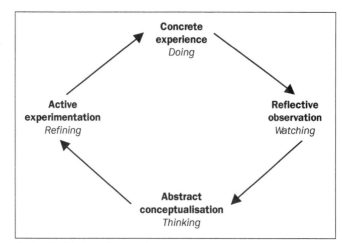

Figure 7.1   Kolb's learning cycle

Gibbs' (1988) reflective cycle is widely used in nurse education (see Figure 7.2). It is essentially a refinement of Kolb's cycle and forms a good template or structure for undertaking reflection and reflective writing.

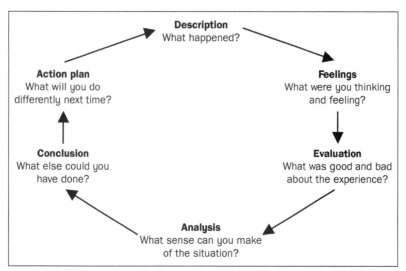

Figure 7.2   Gibbs' reflective cycle

There are also simpler guides to reflection, three of which are addressed below.

Questions that aid reflection

- What happened? (This should be described in as much detail as possible)
- How do I feel about it?
- What was my role?
- Why did I/we do it that way?
- What factors influenced my actions?
- What was the intended outcome? What was I trying to achieve?
- What was the outcome?
- What does the theory say?
- What other ways are there of doing it?
- What can I do differently next time?
- What other skills or knowledge do I need?
- What have I learnt?

INCIDENT short reflection

- What happened?
- Why did it happen?
- How can I change it?

Incident/procedure grid to aid reflection

What went well?	What did not go well?
How could I have done it differently?	What learning do I need to do?

Types of portfolio evidence

The experience of building a portfolio serves as reminder of the process that the students you will be mentoring have to go through. The same types and range of evidence can be used. Whatever the evidence, it should be accompanied by a rationale for its inclusion. This is usually a short description of the relevance and meaning of the evidence or experience, and how it demonstrates the achievement of a competence.

The amount of evidence is largely a matter of personal choice but it should not be too heavy – a portfolio should be portable. The best guidance is that quality is better than quantity and the material should be relevant to the aims of the portfolio. The following are types of evidence student nurses might use and which mentors will have to scrutinise before signing off. These are also the types of evidence mentors can use to support their achievement of the mentor standards.

Reflective writing

This can be related to almost any aspect of the student's experience and can be used to link theory and practice and identify learning needs. It is usually done in relation to an incident or experience that has made a big impression on the student, either good or bad. Many will use a reflective model to do this as discussed above. Reflective writing does not have to be an essay but should be more than a statement or short paragraph if it is to be useful, as it should describe the incident and the student's feelings, as well as analysing it and examining the theory and then drawing out the learning that has taken place. It should then identify further learning needs. Reflective writing can lose its focus if it is too long, which is why some of the simpler models and proformas work well. A typical student will have enough essays to write without adding to the burden. The focus for the mentor when reading or listening to a reflective account is to draw out the learning that has taken place. A 'critical incident analysis' is another such form of reflection but usually goes into greater depth. These analyses and reflections can be presented to the team or colleagues for discussion.

Reflective diary

Reflective diaries are useful because we cannot memorise everything, so it's best to write things up as soon as possible after the event. Many students keep diaries throughout their placements detailing clinical incidents, experiences, and learning. It is helpful for them to do this, as to sit down on week 7 of a placement and try to recall what you have done in the preceding weeks to meet your outcomes is nigh impossible. The diary will be a record of significant events upon which the student can reflect and gather evidence.

Learning contracts

Learning contracts and their assessments, together with the work that went into meeting the objectives of the contract, would make good evidence for a portfolio.

Reflective discussion

Reflective discussion can take place at pre-set times, just after a learning experience or in any spare time available, such as the journey between visits in the community. Such discussions can be useful for identifying the student's knowledge base but also their values and attitudes.

Question and answer

This can be a formal set of written questions provided by the mentor for the student to work on and present back at a later discussion. The student can write the answers and present them as evidence within their portfolio. Less formally, the questions can form the basis of a discussion session between mentor and student, which the student can then write up. It can be even less formal and linked to procedures, with the mentor asking the student 'Why do we do things in a certain way?' or 'How could you do that differently?' This is a good way to assess a student's knowledge base and identify learning needs.

Opinion of others

Testimonials or witness statements can be garnered from others the student has worked with, including nurses other than their mentor, health-care assistants, members of the multidisciplinary team, clients, and carers. Care should be taken with such witness statements or testimonials that the consent of clients and carers was gained. Such testimonials widen the body of opinion as to the student's ability and make the assessment process much more reliable and fair. Such opinion can relate to knowledge, skills, and attitudes, and positive opinions will reinforce the student's position. Witnesses can be asked by the student or their mentor to write a short statement or the student can write a statement about what they have done and how they feel they have performed and ask a witness to sign it.

Direct observation

This relates to direct observation of a student's practice by their mentor. The student will need to record the date and a short description within the portfolio. The observation can be formal or just happen as part of the working day. The mentor would most likely observe the student doing any one thing on several occasions in order to ensure that the level of achievement is consistent. The student's account can vary from a short statement to a reflective piece and be linked to many outcomes.

Articles/leaflets

These can be included as evidence but must be linked to learning outcomes. The student must provide a discussion of their relevance and how they meet the outcomes.

Action plans

Students often draw up an action plan with a mentor early on in the placement if specific learning needs are to be achieved, such as unmet competencies or 'essential skills'. This and its subsequent reviews can form good evidence. It can be linked to theory and show self-awareness and self-direction. Sometimes key skills can be identified, such as drug calculations or injection technique and these can form the basis of an action plan.

Academic work

Occasionally, a piece of academic work can be used as evidence in support of practice experience and as a way of demonstrating the links between theory and practice.

Activity records

Written in a partially reflective style, these are records of activities undertaken such as reassuring a client, accompanying a patient to another department, or organising a pizza night on the mental health ward. There are many activities students undertake that highlight learning and skill but do not fit easily into strict categories.

SWOT analysis

This is covered in detail in Chapter 2, 'The effective mentor', but it is a useful exercise to give to a student. They can undertake an analysis of the learning environment for the team or can analyse their own placement experience or own practice and hence identify future learning needs.

Work-based products

These include anonymous nursing documents such as a nursing report entry, or an assessment or admission the student has undertaken. When linked to other evidence, such as a witness statement from a client, a direct observation by the mentor, and a reflective piece by the student, the whole package will relate to many outcomes. This is a good example of a cluster of high-quality pieces of evidence rather than separate evidence for each outcome.

Insight visits

These are records of a student's visits to other relevant departments or services. The student may include a leaflet outlining the service but should also write about the purpose of the visit, the role the service plays, and the learning they have gained.

Remember to cross-reference and link evidence to the competencies they demonstrate achievement of.

Evidence of achievement of the mentor outcomes

The NMC guidelines for mentor preparation programmes, *Standards to Support Learning and Assessment in Practice* (NMC 2008b), state that they should include at least five days' protected learning time and relevant work-based learning such as mentoring a student under the supervision of an experienced mentor or acting as an associate mentor. This experience itself leads to a plethora of opportunities to provide evidence of achievement of the outcomes.

Examples are provided below of activities and work that can be put forward by budding mentors as evidence of achievement of each of the domains and their outcomes. Usually, there will be various ways of presenting the evidence, such as direct observation or reflective writing; it is up to each student to decide how to present their evidence. Remember that for such things as work products or activities, a short explanation should be provided of how they demonstrate achievement of standards. There will also be much repetition, as many pieces of potential evidence will be relevant to more than one standard. Examples of many of the pieces of evidence quoted here can be found in other chapters.

Evidence

Each of the following boxes relates to one of the NMC mentor domains and cites the clauses within those domains. There then follows a comprehensive list of different activities and forms of evidence a mentor could provide to demonstrate achievement of the NMC mentor competencies. The list is by no means exhaustive, but it is relevant to all nursing specialties and nursing environments. As mentioned earlier, it is the quality not the quantity of evidence that makes a good portfolio.

Domain: Establish effective working relationships

Outcomes

- Demonstrate an understanding of factors that influence how students integrate into practice
- Provide ongoing and constructive support to facilitate transition from one learning environment to another
- Have effective professional and interprofessional working relationships to support learning for entry to the register

Evidence

- Describe and provide evidence of your interprofessional and multidisciplinary role and your teamwork skills
- Describe the value of links with your educational representative from the university and how you might enhance this link in the future
- Understand the local curriculum and student's assessment paperwork
- Describe how you would induct a student into the placement
- Student induction pack/pre-placement welcome letter/placement profile
- Pre-placement student visit protocol
- Importance of and evidence of good communication skills
- Describe how you would welcome a student
- Understand student stress and individual needs
- Protocol for a student's first day, negotiation re: shifts and student's needs
- Protocol for a preliminary interview
- Identify learning needs and develop an initial action plan
- Describe how you will foster associate mentorship for the student
- Importance of recognising the student's level and experience
- Provide teaching appropriate to the level of the learner
- Detail how you will structure feedback and progress interviews and how you provide feedback and support the student
- Student feedback or evaluation of placement
- Students included in team social events

(continued)

- Reflect upon how a new student is supported when they are placed with your area
- Interview students about their experience in your clinical area
- Evidence of your own team working
- Evidence of liaison and working with School of Nursing
- Student's SWOT analysis of your role as a mentor

Domain: Facilitation of learning

Outcomes

- Use knowledge of the student's stage of learning to select appropriate learning opportunities to meet their individual needs
- Facilitate selection of appropriate learning strategies to integrate learning from practice and academic experiences
- Support students in critically reflecting upon their learning experiences in order to enhance future learning

Evidence

- Awareness of student's experience and level of skill and knowledge and competence
- Identify particular needs for a placement
- Identify appropriate learning opportunities
- Identify student's learning style/relevance of learning theories in practice
- Undertake a learning styles inventory
- Maintain student placement resources, e.g. journals, notice board
- Structure opportunity for and facilitate student reflection on practice
- Identify clinical areas for own learning opportunities
- Map learning opportunities to NMC competencies
- Identify creative learning opportunities such as patient pathways
- Use a range of teaching methods with the student
- Provide regular feedback and identify how to make time for students

(continued)

- Familiar with student documentation
- Help the student to write an action plan for their future learning
- Identify relevant insight and multidisciplinary team and specialist staff visits
- Identify teaching sessions, conferences, and meetings the student can attend
- Apply the concept of adult learning
- Encourage student presentations
- Use client feedback as a learning opportunity
- Liaise with link tutor and School of Nursing
- Importance of working with the student on regular basis
- Maximise student direct involvement in patient care
- Concept and value of buddying student with healthcare support workers
- Encourage and act upon student evaluations and feedback of placement
- Maintain students' supernumerary status and work with them at least 40% of the time
- Student's SWOT analysis of your role as a mentor

Domain: Assessment and accountability

Outcomes

- Foster professional growth, personal development, and accountability through support of students in practice
- Demonstrate a breadth of understanding of assessment strategies and the ability to contribute to the total assessment process as part of the teaching team
- Provide constructive feedback to students and assist them in identifying future learning needs and actions. Manage failing students so they may either enhance their performance and capabilities for safe and effective practice or be able to understand their failure and the implications of this for their future

(continued)

- Be accountable for confirming that students have met, or not met, the NMC competencies in practice. As a sign-off mentor confirm that students have met, or not met, the NMC standards of competency in practice and are capable of safe and effective practice

Evidence

- Identify students' main learning needs early and plan assessments

- Identify the level that students are at

- Encourage students to undertake SWOT analysis

- Familiar with assessment paperwork

- Provide formative assessments and constructive feedback, review progress regularly

- Provide examples of assessment interview records (anonymous)

- Provide examples of written feedback/reflection on giving verbal feedback

- Provide an example of an action plan developed with a student (anonymous)

- Provide student with different opportunities to demonstrate competency

- Utilise associate mentors and the opinion of others to improve reliability of assessments

- Students' responsibilities regarding assessment

- Understand assessment biases and barriers to assessment

- Reflect upon how students are assessed in your placement area. What methods are used and are they valid and reliable?

- Understand the range of assessment methods and evidence a student can use

- Identify fair procedures for supporting a student who is not achieving

- Aware of Bloom's taxonomy when assessing students

- Aware of importance of role modelling

- Describe the mentor's accountability relating to assessment

- Documentation and reflection of assessments undertaken

(continued)

- Give due regard to the professional issues of behaviour, enthusiasm, and attitude

- Undertake regular mentor updating

- Liaise with link tutor and School of Nursing

- Managing failing students

Domain: Evaluation of learning

Outcomes

- Contribute to evaluation of student learning and assessment experiences – proposing aspects for change as a result of such evaluation

- Participate in self and peer evaluation to facilitate personal development, and contribute to the development of others

Evidence

- Produce a student evaluation form for the clinical area

- Provide evidence of student evaluations and feedback

- Provide evidence of changes introduced in the light of student feedback

- Provide regular constructive feedback to students

- Provide regular opportunities for reflection

- Student's individual learning needs are identified

- Aware of the range of evidence a student can provide

- Liaise with similar placement areas to share expertise

- Regularly liaise with School of Nursing to support and monitor placement experience

- Read the most recent educational audit of your placement

- Provide examples of assessment interview records (anonymous)

- Provide an example of an action plan developed with a student (anonymous)

- Observe or undertake an educational audit

- SWOT analysis of placement

(continued)

- SWOT analysis of your role as a mentor
- Regular team discussion/reflection regarding student experience
- Maintain evidence-based resources such as journals
- Provide evidence of own continuing professional development
- Show involvement in clinical supervision
- Facilitate regular reflection with the student
- Show that practice reflects current thinking and new evidence is implemented

Domain: Creating an environment for learning

Outcomes

- Support students to identify both learning needs and experiences that are appropriate to their level of learning
- Use a range of learning experiences, involving patients, clients, carers, and the professional team, to meet the defined learning needs
- Identify aspects of the learning environment that could be enhanced – negotiating with others to make appropriate changes
- Act as a resource to facilitate the personal and professional developments of others

Evidence

- Welcoming a student, protocol for first day/placement profile
- Induction/welcome pack and socialisation into clinical team/orientation
- Humanistic approach/communication skills
- Open and democratic team ethos displayed
- Health and safety concerns/processes
- Incident and accident reporting
- Facilitate students; identification of learning needs and an action plan
- Identify students' level and experience
- Reflect upon importance of students' supernumerary status

(continued)

- Reflect upon the mentor's role in motivating students
- Identify with student a range of learning opportunities mapped to competencies
- Maintain student placement resources, such as journals, notice board
- Structure opportunity for and facilitate student reflection on practice
- Demonstrate access to team/in-house training sessions
- Develop a placement-specific workbook for students
- Identify and facilitate insight visits
- Involve healthcare support workers
- Enhance team evidence base
- Understand students' individual needs and possible stressors affecting learning
- Encourage healthcare assistants to be buddies, supporting other mentors
- Demonstrate own continuing professional development and team development
- Show atmosphere encourages students' questions and expression of views
- Evidence of team/associate mentoring
- Evidence of team accessing mentor updates/good links with School of Nursing
- Gather and act upon student feedback of placement experience
- Engage in and act upon educational and clinical audit
- Identify and audit the health and safety aspects of your placement
- Student's SWOT analysis of your role as a mentor

Domain: Context of practice

Outcomes

- Contribute to the development of an environment in which effective practice is fostered, implemented, evaluated, and disseminated

(continued)

- Set and maintain professional boundaries that are sufficiently flexible for providing interprofessional care
- Initiate and respond to practice developments to ensure safe and effective care is achieved and an effective learning environment is maintained

Evidence

- Maintain and enhance team evidence base
- Demonstrate up-to-date practice/continuing professional development
- Adhere to local and national policies and standards
- Demonstrate involvement in educational and clinical audit, quality assurance
- Open/democratic atmosphere that encourages students' questions and views
- Structure opportunity for and facilitate student reflection on practice
- Students helped to access evidence base via resources and time
- Clinical supervision
- Students encouraged to teach and present cases to the team
- Encourage and act upon student feedback
- Reflect upon what makes your area a specialty
- Show constructive use of ward meetings
- Provide evidence of robust complaints procedure and acting upon such
- Research encouraged/engaged in at team level
- Robust links with School of Nursing
- Good interface with public/patient information leaflets
- Importance of attitude, enthusiasm, and professionalism
- Multidisciplinary/interprofessional working
- Journal reading and maintaining currency
- Involvement with practice development
- Clients/carers encouraged to participate in own care
- Health and safety procedures adhered to

Domain: Evidence-based practice

Outcomes

- Identify and apply research- and evidence-based practice to own area of practice
- Contribute to strategies to increase or review the evidence base used to support practice
- Support students in applying an evidence base to their practice area

Evidence

- Robust links with School of Nursing
- Research encouraged/engaged in at team level
- Students helped to access evidence base via resources and time
- Clinical supervision
- Open/democratic atmosphere that encourages students' questions and views
- Evidence of robust complaints procedure and acting upon such
- Demonstrate up-to-date practice/continuing professional development
- Maintain and enhance team evidence base
- Identify deficits in the team's evidence base/changes needed in practice
- Adhere to local and national policies and standards
- Identify a recent change in practice that has enhanced patient care
- Quality assurance and clinical audit
- Local and national standards
- Involvement of specialist nurses/professionals
- Regular team teaching sessions/ward-based clinical discussions
- Provide evidence of staff training and development activity
- Multidisciplinary team working
- Student feedback is gathered and acted upon
- Resources such as journals for staff and students are plentiful and current
- Students encouraged to link theory and practice

(continued)

- SWOT analysis of ward evidence use/resources
- Participation of patients, carers, and the public is encouraged
- Students encouraged to teach and share knowledge
- Describe role of the mentor in relation to evidence-based practice
- Provide an example of a piece of research relevant to your practice and discuss its implications for your practice

Domain: Leadership

Outcomes

- Plan a series of learning experiences that will meet students' defined learning needs
- Be an advocate for students to support them accessing learning opportunities that meet their individual needs involving a range of other professionals, patients, clients, and carers
- Prioritise work to accommodate support of students within their practice
- Provide feedback about the effectiveness of learning and assessment in practice

Evidence

- Be aware of the power of role modelling and the mentor's influence on students
- Importance of good communication skills with both clients and other professionals
- Use evidence-based practice and access up-to-date information
- Demonstrate continuing professional development/best practice
- Adhere to national and local standards and policies
- Demonstrate motivation and enthusiasm, open and approachable
- Identify students' learning needs and helps draw up action plans for such
- Support students' supernumerary status

(continued)

- Develop a week-by-week learning programme for students
- Aware of roles and accountability of mentor
- Good powers of delegation and assertiveness
- Have decision-making and problem-solving skills
- Give time to students, foster reflection, and hold regular reviews with student
- Demonstrate effective time management so that mentor works with students at least 40% of the time
- Facilitate learning experiences and insight visits
- Demonstrate supportive ethos and aware of students' individual needs
- Humanistic, democratic, collaborative, and professional team-working skills
- Involvement in and good links with School of Nursing
- Act as ambassador for the nursing profession
- Actively develop learning resources
- Good teaching skills
- Facilitate and act upon student evaluations
- Engaged in educational audit

Summary

This chapter has:

- Looked at the structure and features of a portfolio
- Examined the importance of reflection as a learning tool
- Described the types of evidence that might be included in a nursing portfolio
- Outlined a range of evidence relevant to the mentor standards

The next chapter examines a range of strategies to support students on placement and also looks at how we can best support those students with disabilities.

Further reading

Carroll, M., Curtis, L., Higgins, A., Nicholl, H., Redmond, R. and Timmins, F. (2002) Is there a place for reflective practice in the nursing curriculum?, *Nurse Education in Practice*, 2(1): 13–20.

Taylor, B. (2006) *Reflective Practice: A guide for nurses and midwives*. Buckingham: Open University Press.

References

Boud, D., Keough, R. and Walker, D. (1985) *Reflection: Turning experience into learning*. London: Kogan Page.

Dion, W. and Smolenski, M. (2008) Why you need an electronic professional portfolio, *American Nurse Today*, 3(9): 13–14.

Fitzgerald, M. and Chapman, Y. (2000) Theories of reflection for learning, in S. Burns and C. Bulman (eds.) *Reflective Practice in Nursing: The growth of the professional practitioner*. London: Blackwell Science.

Gibbs, G. (1988) *Learning by Doing: A guide to teaching learning methods*. Oxford: Oxford Brookes University.

Kolb, D.A. (1984) *Experiential Learning: Experience as the source of learning and development*. Englewood Cliffs, NJ: Prentice-Hall.

McMullen, M., Endacott, R., Gray, M.A., Jasper, M., Miller, C.M., Scholes, J. et al. (2003) Portfolios and assessment of competence: a review of the literature, *Journal of Advanced Nursing*, 41(3): 283–94.

Nursing and Midwifery Council (NMC) (2004) *Standards of Proficiency for Pre-registration Nursing Education*. London: NMC.

Nursing and Midwifery Council (NMC) (2008a) *The PREP Handbook*. London: NMC.

Nursing and Midwifery Council (NMC) (2008b) *Standards to Support Learning and Assessment in Practice: NMC standards for mentors, practice teachers and teachers*, 2nd edn. London: NMC.

Nursing and Midwifery Council (NMC) (2010) *Standards for Pre-registration Nursing Education*. London: NMC. Available at: http://standards.nmc-uk.org/Published-Documents/Standards%20for%20pre-registration%20nursing%20education%2016082010.pdf [accessed 2 March 2014].

Nursing and Midwifery Council (NMC) (2011) *The Prep Handbook*. London: NMC.

Oxford University Press (2005) *Compact Oxford English Dictionary of Current English*, 3rd edn. Oxford: Oxford University Press.

Timmins, F. (2008) *Making Sense of Portfolios: A guide for nursing students*. Maidenhead: Open University Press.

8 Helping students and mentors survive a placement

Key points

- It is important that mentors use associate mentors
- Healthcare support workers can act as a good support mechanism for students
- Disability is not a barrier to becoming a good nurse
- Mentors need to be vigilant for signs of stress in student nurses

NMC (2008) domains and outcomes for a mentor related to this chapter

Establish effective working relationships

- Have effective professional and interprofessional working relationships to support learning for entry to the register
- Provide ongoing and constructive support to facilitate transition from one learning environment to another

Facilitation of learning

- Use knowledge of the student's stage of learning to select appropriate learning opportunities to meet their individual needs
- Support students in critically reflecting upon their learning experiences in order to enhance future learning

Assessment and accountability

- Provide constructive feedback to students and assist them in identifying future learning needs and actions

Creating an environment for learning

- Support students to identify both learning needs and experiences that are appropriate to their level of learning

(continued)

Leadership

- Plan a series of learning experiences that will meet students' defined learning needs

- Be an advocate for students to support them accessing learning opportunities that meet their individual needs – involving a range of other professionals, patients, clients, and carers

- Prioritise work to accommodate support of students within their practice

Support mechanisms other than the mentor

There are support mechanisms other than their mentor that a student can call upon, and it is important that the mentor does not regard the student as 'theirs' alone. Denying the student the opportunity to work with others is detrimental to their learning and renders assessment unnecessarily subjective. A good mentor will draw upon a range of others to support the student in their mentoring role.

Third-year student on accident and emergency department placement

The nurses and healthcare assistants made me feel welcome, everyone let me work alongside them, they encouraged me to participate rather than just observe which was great. Also the receptionists, housekeepers, and porters were always helpful.

Associate mentors

It is educationally good practice to learn from more than one source, and this is a large part of the value of having associate mentors. Students get to see the different ways in which different nurses approach the same situation, and thus witness a wider range of skills, techniques, and problem-solving abilities. It is also the responsibility of the associate mentor to look after the student in the absence of the main mentor, who cannot always be with the student. If a clinical area has a large influx of students, it may be necessary to have a named associate mentor to whom the student can turn. A team mentoring approach can also work but care must be taken to ensure the students are indeed being looked after, and not to assume that someone else is doing it. In relation to assessment, evidence of competence can be drawn from a wider range of sources the more people the student has worked with. This broader range of opinion renders the assessment process much more objective and thus fairer.

Third-year student in an accident and emergency department

Both my mentors were very supportive and encouraging, and gave praise when I did something well. I was made to feel of use and able to contribute. The experience has made me feel more confident about dealing with emergency situations.

Second-year student in an accident and emergency department

Throughout the placement, I felt fully supported and encouraged and very quickly felt a valued member of the team. I thoroughly enjoyed the work undertaken and working with such a professional and knowledgeable team. They all had trust in my abilities, which increased my confidence.

Link tutor/personal tutor

Each student will have a personal tutor from the School of Nursing/university whose role it is to support that student throughout their programme. This tutor will be the main contact for any mentor who has concerns about a student that cannot be resolved between the mentor and the student alone. Similarly, the student can access their personal tutor to discuss placement difficulties. Personal tutors also have a pastoral role and are available to support the student with personal or domestic difficulties as well as academic and practice ones.

University systems for supporting placements have changed over the years but every placement area should have a named educational representative or 'link tutor' whose role it is to monitor and support that placement. They might, for example, help the placement identify specific learning experiences and help map the learning opportunities to competencies. They might meet with students during their placements to monitor their progress and discuss their learning. Such visits are also used to meet with and support mentors and also keep them up to date with any curriculum changes. The link tutor should ensure that their contact details are available in the clinical area. This is especially important for students who are having difficulties on a placement, as they may not wish to discuss them with placement staff. The link tutor will be able to help the student to identify the best way forward and support them in this.

Mentors are crucial to students in demonstrating the practical application of the theory learnt in class and in testing the evidence base. However, it is important that mentors do not offer advice regarding academic matters. Many assignments will be based upon the student's practice experience, and many students will ask for their mentor's advice and help. Mentors can comment upon the practice aspects of a student's assignment but must be careful not to get drawn into the academic aspects and must refer the student back to their tutors.

Fellow students

Being the only student in a clinical area is beneficial in terms of the learning opportunities that arise. However, this can be a lonely experience and most students will prefer to be placed with a colleague from whom they can draw support. Most universities encourage third-year students to support junior students in a 'buddy' role. This gives them the opportunity to develop both their teaching and mentoring skills. Much support can be derived from a third-year student who until only recently was in the same position as their more junior, and less confident, fellow student.

First-year mental health student on admission ward

I found it really daunting at first and I was very nervous. Everyone seemed so in control and professional whereas I hadn't a clue as to what to do and just felt like a fish out of water. I was intimidated by everyone else's ability. I was so glad that the second-year student was on placement with me because he reassured me that he felt exactly the same last year and he showed me the ropes.

Healthcare support worker (HCSW)

The importance of healthcare support workers (also known as healthcare assistants and formerly nursing auxiliaries) in nurse education should not be underestimated. They possess a wealth of skills and experience in caring that they can pass on, as well as providing a support mechanism to students. By formalising and recognising their supportive and educational function, HCSWs can be given an enhanced role, which might help to enhance their status and sense of worth. An HCSW can be allocated to a student in much the same way as students are allocated a mentor. In this way, the student will have another member of staff to call upon. In 'befriending' the student, the HCSW can help show them the ropes and routines. They will be someone whom the student can work alongside and learn the many crucial skills of basic nursing care, such as feeding patients who are unable to feed themselves or explaining patients' observation charts. By carrying out this role and working closely with the student, the HCSW is also in a position to help the mentor by providing feedback on how the student is doing. They can of course also provide the student with witness statements.

Advice for students on placement

New nurse mentors on a recent workshop were asked what advice could be given to students on placement. The following are some of their suggestions:

(continued)

- Research the placement and its learning opportunities
- Organise a short pre-placement visit and pick up a placement welcome/student pack
- Check transport, parking, location, shifts, etc.
- Complete your aims and objectives for the placement to discuss at initial interview
- Be open-minded and positive even if it's not a specialism you like; there is always much you can learn
- Have a willingness to learn and show enthusiasm
- Have a good sense of humour and smile
- Highlight concerns and worries about your placement early
- Be proactive in seeking out learning opportunities and use them wisely
- If you are not sure, ask! In fact, ask questions as much as you can
- Be mindful of good timekeeping and the quality of reliability
- Be professional outside of work as well as inside it
- Make yourself aware of policies and procedures
- Learn to live without your mobile phone for the shift
- Display caring and compassion towards the clients
- Be non-judgemental
- Be respectful of colleagues
- Use the experience of healthcare support workers
- Manage your own learning
- Communicate your learning needs
- Value your own experience
- Present your paperwork/evidence to your mentor on a regular basis

There were also several references to identifying 'preferred choice of biscuit' that I feel allude to the human touch and being prepared to muck in and be part of the team.

HCSW Befriender Scheme – An experience

This scheme was introduced to enhance the level of support provided to students on placement and to develop better relationships between

(continued)

HCSWs and students. It aimed to address tensions between the roles of the students and the support workers on an orthopaedic ward at a small general hospital. These tensions were identified from student evaluations and they suggested a lack of understanding of each other's roles. Questions such as 'who was in charge of who' arose. This was true in particular of more senior students. The support workers were asked to identify which aspects of their role corresponded most closely with those of the students. Three main aspects were identified: orientation, support, and consolidation of basic skills. It was hoped that that by working as a named friend of a student, it would enhance team work and mutual understanding.

Examples of the role include greeting the student on their first day, being involved in their induction to the area, showing them around, advising them where things can be found, advising on tea breaks, and working with them when carrying out a range of basic nursing care. The latter includes a range of activities throughout the patient's journey, such as personal hygiene, toileting and mouth care, preparing patients and their documentation for theatre or investigations, as well as many other clinical skills.

The students provided positive evaluations of their placements, and their relationship with HCSWs was viewed as one of the most valued aspects. In addition, the support workers claimed they felt more valued and confident in their role in supporting students.

(Clare Sobieraj, Nurse Lecturer, University of Nottingham)

First-year student on adult acute ward

The nursing assistants made me feel welcome, as often the other staff were too busy. They showed me how to give the patients personal care. They understood that I hadn't had any ward experience before and took me under their wings. I felt like I learnt a lot just by getting on with the everyday stuff. Each NA [nursing assistant] had a student to orient around the ward for the first couple of shifts not only to teach us but to give them some responsibility.

Second-year student on an emergency assessment unit placement

I found the unit quite intimidating in the first few weeks given the extreme nature of the unit, but the NAs were great – they helped me through and got me settled.

The students' own responsibility

It is important that the mentor meet with the student as early in their placement as possible, when the mentor can set clear goals and highlight the student's responsibilities in relation to the placement and the mentor. Such responsibilities will include timekeeping and other professional issues alongside the student's responsibility to present the mentor with robust evidence on a frequent basis, thus keeping their paperwork up to date. The student has a responsibility to flag up any problems and issues as early as possible. The student must also be made aware that they are responsible for their own learning; they need to identify their particular learning needs and ways of meeting them and if necessary present an action plan for these.

How not to do it!

First-year mental health student on mental health ward for the elderly

Some of the staff could have been more friendly. There should be more opportunity for first years to do things rather than just letting the third-year students do all the main work. It would have been good to be shown more things such as the paperwork. But this was always given to third years on their final placements and I was forgotten about.

Second-year student on surgical ward

We should have been given more opportunities . . . it was difficult to fit into the established team, it felt uncomfortable working with some staff. We were there to learn but sometimes I felt we were just 'running errands' for others.

Students with disabilities and difficulties

Disabilities and health conditions are addressed during the initial selection process when students apply to do their training. Having been accepted upon a course, some assume that it has been agreed that the disability is no barrier to becoming a competent nurse. However, some disabilities are only recognised for the first time once a student's training has begun.

Disability

Disability, reasonable adjustments, non-disclosure, and the mentor's role

The Royal College of Nursing subscribes to the social model of disability and is committed to disability equality. According to The Equality Act 2010, a person has a disability if:

- They have a physical or mental impairment

- The impairment has a substantial and long-term adverse affect on their ability to perform normal day-to-day activities

Examples include:

- physical impairments

- sensory impairments

- specific learning difficulties (e.g. dyslexia)

- mental health conditions

- long-term conditions

Under the Act, it is unlawful for individuals to be treated less favourably as a result of their disability.

A potential nursing student has the opportunity to declare a health condition and/or disability on the UCAS application form. If a student declares a disability, various assessments will be undertaken. An applicant with a health issue will have an assessment by an occupational health team, whose job it is to determine if they are fit to undertake the course. Most universities offer in-house student support in the form of disability advice and assessments. Once a disability is diagnosed, an assessment is undertaken to determine whether reasonable adjustments can put in place while the student is in university and on placement.

Reasonable adjustments

The duty to make reasonable adjustments is detailed in the Disability Discrimination Act 2005.

It is the university's academic and support staff's responsibility to ensure they fulfil their duty to make anticipatory adjustments to the teaching, learning, and assessment process. When a student is on placement, mentors have a duty to ensure adjustments are in place. The Nursing and Midwifery Council states that their concern is whether an adjustment enables a nurse to achieve 'safe and effective practice without supervision' (NMC 2010).

(continued)

Factors to consider when deciding if an adjustment is reasonable include:

- the need to maintain academic and practice competence standards
- the financial cost of the adjustment and the resources available
- the practicality of the adjustment
- the effectiveness of the adjustment
- the health and safety of the student, patients, fellow students, and placement staff

Examples of realistic adjustments for a student in placement include:

- A student with diabetes: a mentor needs to ensure they are able to take regular meal breaks and access their medication.
- A student with dyslexia: is the student able to use a colour overlay on paper?

The non-disclosing student

There is no legal requirement for an individual to disclose a disability even if it is known. Many students do not see themselves as disabled, or may not want to disclose a disability for fear of repercussions and stigma. Academic staff should encourage a student to disclose their disability to their mentor. Any disclosure needs to be treated confidentially and only shared with the placement team with the student's consent. Without disclosure the placement is unable to put in place any adjustments.

The diagnosis of a disability may be made while a student is on placement and only become apparent as a consequence of the student's experiences. For example, a student who finds it difficult to retain new information may have developed self-managing strategies for their dyslexia by taking notes and now find they can't cope.

A mentor may be the first to recognise a struggling student and be best placed to encourage them to access study support and inform the university's academic staff.

Role of the mentor

While working with a student, a mentor needs to develop a relationship in which the student feels safe to disclose a disability. The mentor then needs to consider what if any reasonable adjustments the placement can provide to support the student in their learning. With the student's consent, it should be documented in the student's placement record. A mentor might suspect a disability like dyslexia and make their suspicions known to the student. A mentor may need to contact academic staff for guidance and support.

(Chris Craggs, Senior Lecturer in Nursing, University of Lincoln)

NMAS statistics

The Nursing and Midwifery Admissions Service (NMAS) (now defunct, as all admissions go through UCAS, the university clearing system) used to collect statistics relating to disability among nursing applicants and those accepted onto nursing courses. The last statistics relating to 2007 show that of 12,763 applicants accepted onto nursing courses, those with a disability were as follows:

Learning disability	323
Blind/partially sighted	20
Deaf/partial hearing	48
Wheelchair mobility	11
Mental health	55
Unseen disability	104
Multiple disabilities	13
Other disability	97
Not known	572

(*Source*: http://www.nmas.ac.uk/)

What this tells us is that roughly 10% had some form of disability. So nursing students with disabilities are by no means rare and we can be fairly sure the true figures were higher, as it is likely that some applicants would not have disclosed their disability through fear of rejection from the course.

Mentors can also encourage students to access university disability liaison officers to explore the services and help they can offer.

Dyslexia

The British Dyslexia Association (BDA) defines dyslexia as a specific learning difficulty that mainly affects the development of literacy and language-related skills. The Parliamentary Office of Science and Technology (2004) suggest that the prevalence of dyslexia is between 2% and 15% of the UK population.

There are many variations and forms of dyslexia and thus no one adequate definition. Simply defined, it is difficulty with reading and writing. The BDA suggest that it is characterised by difficulties with processing speech and the written word, memory, and the speed at which we process information. It can also be indicated by poor handwriting and spelling alongside poor time management and organisational skills. It is usually resistant to conventional teaching methods but, as the BDA point out, its effects can be offset with the help of information technology and support.

Difficulties dyslexic students may face in practice

- Reading and writing up reports, filling in forms
- Poor time management/prioritising workload
- Poor hand–eye coordination/difficulty with certain practical procedures
- Remembering the steps of a complex procedure or all the points made at a handover

Often in the case of dyslexia, 'reasonable adjustments' can be made, including:

- going over explanations several times/repeating instructions;
- using a tape-recorder/taking notes;
- allowing extra time to complete tasks and write things up;
- providing reminders and encouraging the use of lists;
- using coloured paper for handouts/using a highlighter;
- backing up multiple instructions for complicated procedures with flow charts or diagrams;
- giving reading material out in advance;
- providing extra teaching and support;
- allowing more flexibility with working hours;
- using a wall planner to help with organisational problems and meeting deadlines;
- providing a glossary of terms commonly used on the placement;
- giving practical demonstrations to back up verbal explanations.

The Royal College of Nursing (RCN 2007), in a toolkit for mentors, offers sound practical advice, such as allowing students to practise writing up notes in rough before committing them to the documentation. Mentors can also help by encouraging the student to access help through the British Dyslexia Association and the university's academic support or disability liaison departments.

While reasonable adjustments can be made to help a student with dyslexia, they still have to demonstrate that they are fit to practise and meet all the NMC competencies. Thus the mentor needs to help the student overcome their difficulties rather than avoid them. It is important to remember that all dyslexic students will be different and have varied needs and what works for one student might not necessarily work for the next.

Dyscalculia

This condition affects the ability to work with numbers and thus perform calculations, something that is very important in nursing in relation to medication. Mentors should encourage the use of calculators to check calculations and allow students extra time. Mentors must check the accuracy of students' calculations and get students to show them how they arrived at the result. This will help pinpoint what aspects of the calculation are proving difficult, and whether extra support and tuition is appropriate.

Sickness and stress

European law dictates that student nurses have to complete a set number of hours before they are eligible to register. Because of this students are often reluctant to declare sickness for fear of having to make up time later on a subsequent placement or at the end of their course. Most nurse education programmes allow for some sick days so that students don't undertake more placement hours than the legal requirement. Compared with other higher education courses and many degrees, nurse training is a comparatively stiff undertaking. The combination of educational and professional qualification means that students may well have several assignments ongoing and be working full time in the clinical area as well as balancing these demands with a social and domestic life. Mentors can help by passing on time management skills. Mentors need to be aware of the physical health of students and encourage them to take time out if necessary. A sick or overtired nurse is a dangerous nurse and the ethics and accountability of ploughing on regardless might be usefully explored with students. Mentors should also point out to students the sickness policy and ensure the student is aware of their obligation to notify the School of Nursing and placement. Students should also be made aware that they should complete a self-certificate if the sickness is for more than three consecutive days, and a certificate from their GP will be required if they are off for more than eight days.

There are many reasons why a student might suffer undue stress while on placement: they may be overloaded with assignments, have family and personal problems, be a first-year student not familiar with the healthcare environment or a third-year student worried about their imminent qualification – they may also be having a hard time on a placement for a variety of reasons. The most important thing is that the mentor meets the mentor standard 'Establishing effective working relationships'. Such a mentor will have developed an open and friendly relationship with their student, who will feel that they are approachable and someone with whom they can share their worries without fear of criticism.

Second-year mental health student

Here I was allowed to be a student and never classed in the numbers; this enabled me to learn more effectively and have more time to gain the experience I needed. The team were especially good, as I had to have some time out due to personal issues, but they were very supportive and recognised that I was under some stress. My mentor in particular took the time to make sure I was OK.

Mentors need to be alert to the signs of stress and offer the student support. They also need to be familiar with workplace and university support systems such as counselling services as well as the student's personal tutor.

Signs that may be indicative of stress in students

- Absence
- Lateness/poor timekeeping
- Underperformance
- Lack of motivation
- Tiredness
- Poor concentration
- Emotional/agitated/irritable
- Withdrawn and quiet
- Physical illness/aches, pains, colds, etc.
- Poor sleep and diet
- Behavioural changes

Mentors may also advise that students seek help from occupational health departments or put them in touch with professional organization helplines, such as that of the Royal College of Nursing.

Workplace harassment

In its worst form, this is bullying and can range from physical violence to more subtle forms of psychological or sexual harassment. A good mentor will be one the student feels they can approach if they suffer harassment from other staff or clients. A good mentor will also pick up on the signs that something is amiss, such as changes in the student's behaviour similar to those relating to stress. Mentors should support students through the process of reporting such incidents to the School of Nursing and the healthcare trust, and ensure that they are protected from further harassment. A discussion between mentor and student could be had on the ethics and duty to report such incidents, since reporting is a means of protecting others from being harassed. The mentor should also point out that a staff member who bullies students could also be taking advantage of clients. Increasingly nurses are exposed to bullying and harassment from clients. Sometimes this is the result of the patient's illness and can thus be put into context and tolerated to a degree, but in can occur, for example, as the result of an alcohol-fuelled incident in a busy accident and emergency department. In areas where such incidents are commonplace, mentors should go through the local policy with students in relation to prevention of abuse, self-protection, and the reporting procedure and support mechanisms.

Bad practice

At some stage in their training, students will almost inevitably witness practices that they believe to be poor or even unsafe. Their interpretation of events may be due to a lack of understanding of the context of the practice or the individual client's needs and preferences. The approachable mentor will be able to encourage the student to question practices they do not understand or might not agree with, and hold an open discussion around the issues. Occasionally, however, a student will witness bad practice that does need to be reported, and a good relationship with the mentor will usually facilitate this process, the mentor again discussing the incident and guiding the student through the reporting process, being both supportive and protective of the student. The mentor will have to call upon their professionalism here, as it will often be one of their colleagues about whom the allegation is made. The mentor could also remind the student about adult protection issues and inform them of the local adult protection service, its contact details and reporting procedures.

Mentors' guide to surviving a placement!

- **Spread the load.** Utilise associate mentors, HCSWs, senior students, and the rest of the multidisciplinary team. This reduces the burden on you, gives the student wider experience of seeing how different people work, and makes the assessment much fairer and more objective. It also enhances the role of the HCSW.

- **Early interview.** Interview the student early in the placement to ascertain their level of competence. This also allows you to inform the student of their responsibilities towards you and their own learning.

(continued)

- **Use insight visits.** These give the student more experience and you time out.

- **Identify issues early on.** The longer you leave a problem, the harder it becomes to sort out.

- **Share problems.** If you consider the student a potential failure, have a tripartite interview between you, the student, and their tutor.

- **Develop a relationship with the link tutor.** Such tutors are a good source of support and it is advantageous already to have a close working relationship when things go wrong.

- **Maintain strong professional boundaries.** Becoming too friendly with the student makes it harder to be critical (in the positive sense) and objective.

- **Be enthusiastic.** The less enthusiastic you are, the more likely it is the student will adopt the same attitude.

- **Make time.** Be strict about this and assertive with managers and other staff to protect your time with students. The risk of not doing so is to eat into your own time.

- **Make the student responsible.** Ensure the student takes responsibility for their own learning by getting them to identify what they want to achieve, write their own action plans, organize insight visits, and book times to meet with you to go over their evidence and documentation. Make them responsible for convincing you they are meeting their outcomes.

- **Meet regularly.** Regularly reviewing progress means you will not have to sit down for a lengthy session going through evidence. Do it weekly, if not more frequently.

- **Give constructive feedback.** Clear, honest, and actionable feedback will make life easier for both of you.

Summary

This chapter has:

- Examined the support systems available for students

- Described the valuable role support workers can play

- Detailed mechanisms for supporting students with disabilities

- Discussed how to support the student under stress

- Examined sources of support for the mentor

Having taught and assessed our students, we obviously hope they achieve their competencies and go on to become excellent nurses. However, not all students will do so.

We now turn our attention to failing students. The next chapter explores how best to manage and support a student who is not performing well and looks at why nurses are traditionally reluctant to fail students, sometimes to the detriment of the profession.

Further reading

Royal College of Nursing (RCN) (2002) *Helping Students Get the Best from Their Practice Placements: A Royal College of Nursing toolkit.* London: RCN.

Royal College of Nursing (RCN) (2007) *Guidance for Mentors of Student Nurses and Midwives: An RCN toolkit.* London: RCN. This is a toolkit designed by the Royal College to assist mentors in their role and outlines the responsibilities of the mentor and those of the student. It looks at what constitutes an effective practice placement and addresses mentoring students with special needs and the support available for mentors.

Storr, H., Wray, J. and Draper, P. (2011) Supporting disabled student nurses from registration to qualification: a review of United Kingdom (UK) literature, *Nurse Education Today*, 31(8): 29–33.

White, J. (2007) Supporting nursing students with dyslexia in clinical practice, *Nursing Standard*, 21(19): 35–42.

Useful web resources

www.bdadyslexia.org.uk
This is the website of the British Dyslexia Association, which exists to help those with dyslexia reach their potential. It has very good information sources and useful links.

www.legislation.gov.uk/ukpga/2010/15/contents
This is a link to the full text of the Equality Act 2010. A summary is available at: https://www.gov.uk/government/uploads/system/uploads/attachment_data/file/85017/individual-rights1.pdf

http://www.direct.gov.uk/en/DisabledPeople/RightsAndObligations/DisabilityRights
This is a very useful site with links to the Disability Discrimination Acts.

www.equalityhumanrights.com/
The Equality and Human Rights Commission superseded the Disability Rights Commission in October 2007 and has a wealth of information in relation to disability.

www.beingdyslexic.co.uk and www.dyslexiaaction.org.uk
These are two other excellent sites with much useful information and guidance regarding making adjustments in the workplace.

www.elderabuse.org.uk
This is the Action on Elder Abuse site and despite the name, it relates to common issues of 'adult' protection and is very useful and informative, looking at how to recognise abuse and what to do about it.

References

Nursing and Midwifery Council (NMC) (2008) *Standards to Support Learning and Assessment in Practice: NMC standards for mentors, practice teachers and teachers*, 2nd edn. London: NMC.

Nursing and Midwifery Council (NMC) (2010) *Good Health and Good Character Guidance for Students, Nurses and Midwives*. London: NMC. Available at: www.nmc-uk.org/Students/Good-Health-and-Good-Character-for-students-nurses-and-midwives/Reasonable-adjustments/ [accessed 2 March 2014].

Parliamentary Office of Science and Technology (2004) *Dyslexia and Dyscalculia*. Postnote No 226. Available at: http://www.parliament.uk/briefing-papers/POST-PN-226/ dyslexia-and-dyscalculiajuly-2004 [accessed 12 March 2014].

Royal College of Nursing (RCN) (2007) *Guidance for Mentors of Student Nurses and Midwives: An RCN toolkit*. London: RCN.

9 Supporting failing students

Key points

- Evidence suggests that nurses are reluctant to fail students for a variety of reasons

- Good feedback is a key skill in supporting students

- There is a clear and fair process for supporting a failing student

- Assessing a student's attitude is often overlooked or avoided but there are sound mechanisms for doing so

- It is important to recognise that support systems for students are also support systems for mentors

NMC (2008a) domains and outcomes for a mentor related to this chapter

Establish effective working relationships

- Have effective professional and interprofessional working relationships to support learning for entry to the register

- Provide ongoing and constructive support to facilitate transition from one learning environment to another

Facilitation of learning

- Support students in critically reflecting upon their learning experiences in order to enhance future learning

Assessment and accountability

- Provide constructive feedback to students and assist them in identifying future learning needs and actions. Manage failing students so they may either enhance their performance and capabilities for safe and effective practice, or be able to understand their failure and the implications of this for their future

(continued)

- Be accountable for confirming that students have met, or not met, the NMC competencies in practice. As a sign-off mentor, confirm that students have met, or not met, the NMC standards of competence in practice and are capable of safe and effective practice

Evaluation of learning

- Contribute to evaluation of student learning and assessment experiences – proposing aspects for change as a result of such evaluation

Reflection on failure

Think back to when you had to let someone know they had failed something or had not done very well. If you have never had to do this, think about the last time you gave someone some bad news.

- How did you do it and what would you do differently if you had to do it again?

- What are the important things to get right when doing this?

Reasons for failure

The reasons why a student might fail a placement are not quite as obvious as they might at first seem. Alongside a lack of knowledge and poor, unsafe clinical skills, the evidence suggests that many students fail for 'professional' reasons. Duffy and Hardicre (2007) identify a range of reasons from the literature to indicate that a student may be failing that have little to do with clinical competence or knowledge, namely:

- Lack of insight, poor self-awareness, and unresponsive to feedback

- Lack of interest, motivation, enthusiasm or commitment

- Poor communication/interpersonal skills

- Frequently late or absent

- Poor professional behaviour/boundaries

- Preoccupation with personal issues

- Under- or over-confidence

Often these issues are overlooked or at worst ignored in student assessment. Why this is so and what we can do to rectify it is explored in the rest of this chapter.

Dilemma

A first-year student nurse appears to be uninterested in basic nursing care and just wants to deal with acute situations, 'office work', and arrange insight visits. It is his second week with the team. What would be your advice at the next meeting you have with him?

The error of leniency: why mentors fail to fail students!

There has been much emphasis recently on mentors being reluctant to fail nursing students and the repercussions this has for the profession. The main body of evidence stems from a study by Duffy (2003). Duffy examined work by Watson and Harris (1999) in Scotland, which suggested that student nurses were being allowed to pass their clinical placements without demonstrating competence. To determine why this was the case, Duffy undertook a fresh study of 26 mentors and 14 lecturers in Scotland. While this is not a large sample, it does shed light on some important areas of concern. The work of Duffy and others suggests the following reasons for not failing students:

- **Leaving it too late.** Mentors left it until too late in the placement to indicate that there was a problem with the student. This meant that there was not sufficient time to allow the student to do anything about it and thus they were allowed to pass. It is arguably morally wrong to inform a student that they are failing when there is too little time for them to do anything about it.

- **Too early in the nurse's training.** Some mentors were unwilling to fail a student early on in their training, feeling that they hadn't been given enough opportunity to prove themselves or that they would eventually pick up the skills later in their training as they progressed.

- **Too late in the training.** Other mentors felt that it was somehow unfair to fail a student so close to them becoming qualified.

Experienced mentor's reflective discussion with novice mentor

Confidence issues are the commonest difficulties facing students, many of which have not been picked up on previous placements. This makes it difficult to broach the subject of failure with the student, who, naturally, will point out that no concerns have been highlighted in previous placements.

- **Personal consequences.** Some mentors worried about the consequences failure would have for students, not wanting to end their careers or have them removed from the course.

- **External factors.** Some mentors were concerned about the stresses mature students were under, including family commitments, being a carer, and financial responsibilities. These factors swayed mentors to be lenient in relation to assessment.

- **Fear of failing.** Some mentors lack the confidence or assertiveness and find it difficult personally to fail a student.

- **Personal failure.** Some mentors felt it was a personal reflection upon them: a personal failure for not being a good enough mentor.

- **Lack of support.** Some mentors did not fail students because they felt unsupported by tutors of problem students. The tutors were offering advice to these mentors but little in the way of support and were not always available when needed.

- **Lack of time.** Mentors with limited time to work with students because they were too busy with clients were often lenient with students who were borderline. Also, many of the placements, especially in the first year, were too short for the mentor to make a reasonable assessment.

- **Benefit of doubt/error of leniency.** If mentors were in doubt about a student's performance, they were likely to pass them, especially if they hadn't spent much time with them due to pressure of work. Anecdotal evidence suggests that this is a frequent occurrence.

- **Scraping through.** Mentors sometimes recognise students' weaknesses but feel they haven't done badly enough to fail. The suggestion is that mentors only fail students when they are consistently poor.

- **Ignoring attitude.** The evidence suggests that mentors find it hardest to fail students on grounds of attitude. Deficits in knowledge and skills are easier to identify and describe. It is harder to discuss a problem relating to someone's 'attitude'. This is discussed below in greater detail.

- **Lack of documented evidence.** Some lecturers bemoaned the fact that at times there is little written evidence of concern about a student and this contributes to not having enough grounds on which to fail them.

- **Not the mentor's role.** Some mentors felt that it was the job of the School of Nursing or the tutors to fail students. Mentors should merely highlight deficiencies, not fail students.

- **Confusing documentation.** This a common feature of mentor feedback, suggesting that the documentation is not easy to use or understand. Also, many clinical areas take students from different nursing schools and courses, each of which has different documentation. Perhaps the NMC ought introduce a single, national document.

Providing feedback

Providing feedback is a vitally important aspect of supporting a student. The following are good practice guidelines for providing effective feedback.

Toxic feedback!

A good way of learning how to do something well is by identifying how to do it badly.

List the worst possible things you could do when providing feedback to a student when they have not performed well.

Failed second-year mental health student

It was awful. From day one I knew it would be hard work with the mentor not being very pleased at having to have a student. But I didn't expect to be treated so dismissively at the end. No one had said I was doing anything wrong, so when at the final interview she refused to sign me off for some of my competencies I was shocked. I thought I was doing okay, otherwise surely they should have told me. But it was more the manner in which it was done. She said I was too quiet and reserved and that I made clients feel awkward. I admit it is a fault and one I am working on, I do need more confidence. But she just told me I lacked social skills and couldn't relate to people. No other explanation was given and no advice on how to improve was offered, she just got it over as quick as possible. She stood up and said, 'you'll have to discuss it with your tutor' and left.

Good feedback is fundamental to aiding the development of learners. Yet it is an area many mentors are uncomfortable with and, as we have seen, poor feedback has played a large part in the evidence relating to failing to fail. Telling someone what they could do better without eroding their confidence is a skilled task. The following are key aspects of good practice when providing feedback:

- **Feedback should be positive.** Good feedback highlights strengths as well as things giving cause for concern. Use what is called the 'sandwich' technique – areas for improvement are discussed in between positive bits of feedback – as this will ensure the session both begins and ends on a positive note. The areas for improvement should be fed back in terms of constructive and practical ways forward. The student should have a clear idea of exactly what is required of them and how to achieve it. In this way, the student should go away happy, willing to work on the constructive feedback they have received. The non-verbal communication skills of the mentor are important here also, as conveying a positive message relies as much upon posture, eye contact, and tone of voice as the words used. Relating this back to theory, we can see that Skinner's (1971) behaviourist principles are at play here in that positive reinforcement will likely lead to repetition of good skills.

Third-year student on accident and emergency placement

I didn't have an intermediate interview but my co-mentor found the time to do it in my final week. The final interview consisted of my mentor criticising my outcome evidence, she gave no verbal praise or feedback, and her comments were written without discussion.

- **Feedback should be balanced.** Positive feedback also makes people feel good, and giving the student positive feedback will help your working relationship with them and make them feel more at ease, encouraging them to engage more with the clinical work and team. However, if you are never critical when the need arises, the danger is that you will enter into a nice, cosy, uncritical, and thus unhelpful relationship with the student. Such a relationship will make for an easy-going placement but it will be of little value educationally and the student will not learn much. A too cosy relationship can also make it very difficult to be critical when the professional need arises. The feedback needs to focus upon the aspects the student needs to improve upon, sandwiched, of course, between feedback relating to positive aspects of their performance. A good mentor is someone the student respects and they regard as fair, so that they welcome the mentor's opinion and constructive criticism and are able to learn from it. Being able to give constructive criticism in a positive way is a key mentoring skill.

- **Feedback should be timely and expected.** Feedback is most effective if it is given as near to the event that occasioned it as possible. The longer you leave it, the less impact and importance the message will have. Given instantly the feedback is perceived as being highly important: 'It can't be that bad or they would have told me straight away'! If a parent rebukes a child later in the day sometime after the incident, it is a minor issue for the child, but if a parent berates them at the time of the offence, it's a big issue. Feedback given when working alongside a mentor can be instant, but much feedback will be pre-arranged in the form of structured meetings. These should be agreed well in advance so that the student can prepare for them. Unexpected feedback, however, can have a significant impact also.

First-year student on an outpatient clinic placement . . . unexpected feedback

I was a bit embarrassed really, I was just using a quiet time to put some things away and tidy up the dressings trolley and cupboards when my mentor came up to me and said, 'That's really good just getting on with that, it's the sort of thing most people ignore and think someone else will do. I just wanted to tell you that you are doing well and that the rest of the team and patients all tell me the same, so well done.' Then she left and got on with her work. I thought 'wow, what a nice thing'.

- **Feedback should be open, honest, and objective.** This might appear obvious, but feedback should reflect the mentor's observations of a student's behaviour together with the views of co-mentors and other team members – or 'team mentoring' in short. The appeal that 'The mentor didn't like me' or 'We had a personality clash' can be avoided by the adoption of team mentoring and associate mentors. Ensure that the information you base opinions on is both valid and reliable. Openness can be achieved by inviting students to discuss your comments. Such a willingness to enter into a dialogue will often defuse difficult situations and encourage exploration of the issue. If there is a disagreement, acknowledge the other's views and don't get drawn into an argument.

- **Feedback should be thorough.** There is nothing quite so discouraging and annoying as to fail an assessment and be told briefly with little in the way of feedback. Feedback needs to be comprehensive in recognition of the assumed effort the student has made. When a student fails an assessment, the feedback should detail why and what needs to be done to turn their training around. When a student has done well, the feedback should again indicate why and help the student move forwards by highlighting further areas of learning.

- **Feedback should be clear and specific.** By this I mean understandable – 'Don't beat around the bush', 'Tell it like it is', 'Give it to them straight', these are all phrases which deliver the same message. Be precise and to the point, so that the student is under no illusions as to what they must do to improve. Being vague will not help them to identify what went wrong. For example, it is better to say, 'You didn't wash your hands after you opened the dressing pack and so touched the sterile field with dirty hands', than to say, 'You compromised the sterile field'. To reduce the anxiety of a student who has failed an assessment, it is important that you rebuild their confidence by starting their recovery with small, achievable goals.

- **Feedback needs to be motivating.** Too much negativity or feedback that is exclusively bad will serve only to destroy any enthusiasm and motivation the student had left. There are always positives to be found.

- **Feedback should be private.** Ensure that the environment is private and that you will be undisturbed. Let others know that you are not to be disturbed and put a notice on the door.

- **Feedback should be unhurried.** Timetable the meeting into your day and again make others aware that you will not be available at this time. Most students will be anxious and will want to ask questions in an unpressured environment. When delivering bad news to a student, the mentor must put aside their own feelings of discomfort and give the student the time to explore the full meaning and consequences of their poor performance.

- **Feedback should invite self-assessment.** Asking the student's own view of their performance is very useful and opens up a dialogue. It can also avoid an awkward situation for the mentor, as students often identify their own shortcomings. In this way, the mentor is not left with the often unenviable task of highlighting them. Mentors could devise self-assessment tools for students related to their own specific clinical areas and the learning outcomes therein. The student could be asked to work through these and talk through it at their assessment meeting as a way of opening proceedings.

- **Good feedback invites feedback.** The student should always be given the opportunity to comment upon the assessments being made of them. 'How do you feel about what I have just said; do you agree with my view on how you handled the situation?' Inviting feedback will also ensure that the student understands exactly what is required of them.

- **Feedback should be recorded.** This is important on several counts. If the mentor should become ill, or go on nights or annual leave (a common feature of student placement evaluations), or change clinical areas, then a lack of paperwork detailing what has been achieved and what requires attention could cause real problems, with the student having to be reassessed by a new mentor. It is also an excuse for passing an incompetent student through lack of evidence. It is crucial that evidence of what is being failed is recorded together with an action plan for turning this around. This is elaborated upon below.

Second-year student . . . feeling part of it!

One of the nicest compliments I was paid was simply being asked to join the staff on a night out. I really felt that I was part of the team then.

Avoiding failure and failing with fairness

As we have already noted, to set the tone for the placement and get off on the right foot, it is crucial the mentor and student meet early on in the placement. The mentor needs to gain an understanding of the student's level of competence as well as identifying particular learning needs. The following questionnaire can help to achieve this.

First-week questionnaire for students

Here are five simple but searching questions for the student to reflect upon in their first week and discuss with you at the start of week 2:

1. What are your learning objectives for this placement?

2. What do you want to get out of this experience given the specialty we are?

3. What will you do to ensure you do not fail this placement?

4. How will you demonstrate enthusiasm and motivation even if you would never consider this specialty as a career option?

5. What have you got to learn from us?

Questions 2 and 5 are relatively similar but ask the question in a different way.

Such a questionnaire is designed to foster reflection and negate failure especially in regard to attitude.

This section is about how to support a student who is failing and how to manage the process fairly and objectively. It addresses the issue of supporting mentors through this sometimes difficult and always disappointing process.

The failing student

A student nurse who is on placement with you is clearly failing to meet their outcomes halfway through the placement. How would you manage this scenario to help the student turn the situation around?

Students fail placements for a variety of reasons, but certain key factors can help to minimise such an occurrence. The basics of good mentoring must be adhered to and one golden rule relates to the importance of the first and early days of a student's placement. That you meet with and form a good relationship with the student early on is crucial. The student needs to feel welcomed and wanted to fit into the placement quickly and so get on with meeting their competencies. As a mentor, you will also quickly need to appraise the competence of the student to determine what you can let them do and the level of supervision you must supply.

A golden rule

Get to know your student and the level they are at early on.

To pass a placement successfully and achieve competencies, the student cannot afford to leave things in the placement. It is the responsibility of the mentor to ensure that they give the student regular reviews and feedback to ensure that they keep on top of meeting their learning objectives. As we said earlier, it is unfair to 'drop' failure upon the student if we have not previously highlighted their deficiencies.

Duffy (2003) cited several reasons for students failing but the key aspect was the lack of a good mentor/student relationship. Given a good relationship, most potential problems can be resolved.

Managing the process of failure

Managing the process of assessment and feedback is important if the student is to rectify a deficit that could potentially result in failure, and also crucial to objectivity if the student does not manage to overcome the deficit. This process can be broken down into clear stages.

- **Early detection.** Meet with the student early on to discuss their lack of progress. It is usually fairly obvious early on in a placement if a student is not performing at the desired level or is falling short in achieving certain competencies. We can all probably recall instances in many aspects of our lives when we were aware early on of something and alarm bells began to ring but nothing was done about it until it was too late. This should not happen to students on placements. Mentors must meet with students regularly in order to pick up on and feed back potential problems or deficits. It could be viewed as morally wrong to inform a student towards the end of their placement that they have failed. It is wrong on two counts: we did not identify the deficit and we did not give the student sufficient time or guidance to do anything about it.

- **Meet regularly.** The mentor should meet with the student on a frequent and regular basis throughout the placement to discuss progress and monitor achievement of outcomes. It is only through such regular meetings and working with the student sufficiently often that the mentor will become aware of deficits at an early stage. Remember that a student won't necessarily flag his or her own perceived deficits, and occasionally a poor student will successfully navigate a placement undetected because of the lack of close monitoring.

- **Identify deficits and learning needs.** Having identified a deficit or potential area of non-achievement of outcomes, there should be an honest and open discussion as to exactly what the deficit is. Learning needs should then be identified, and an action plan should be agreed upon that states exactly what the student has to do to turn things around.

- **Be objective and supported.** If there are concerns early on in the placement and the mentor has highlighted a deficit that is not being overcome, then the subsequent mid-placement interview should be formalised. To improve objectivity, the mentor should call upon the views of colleagues who have acted as associate mentors. This avoids a failing student blaming their difficulties on a personality clash or that the mentor simply did not like them. To support the mentor, the 'link tutor' or relevant contact from the School of Nursing or university should be invited to take part in the mid-placement interview. This shares the responsibility and supports the mentor, but also ensures it is a fair process for the student. It helps to avoid any ambiguity when, later on, the student's progress is reassessed. This tripartite meeting allows the mentor to express their view and allows the student to give their assessment of the situation in what should be an honest, open, and above all constructive discussion. If it is necessary to invite the link tutor, the student should be made aware of this beforehand and that the meeting will be to discuss their lack of progress and any others concerns the mentor might have. This gives the student a chance to prepare and consider their own view of their progress prior to the meeting. It might be that the student wishes to have independent support at the meeting and this should be encouraged.

- **Be frank, open, and honest.** At the meeting, the mentor should state clearly what exactly the problem is. The student should be encouraged to give their version of events. Usually a shared conclusion can be reached with agreement on the issues. The link tutor can help to broker this.

- **Action plan.** From this meeting, clear agreement should be reached as to what exactly the deficit is or what outcomes are not being met. An action plan should be developed indicating what it is the student has to do to achieve these outcomes. The action plan should also identify what support the student requires and what the mentor and others can do to help the student succeed. The action plan should also set deadlines for achievement and review dates. This should be written down and a copy kept by everyone attending the meeting (i.e. mentor, student, and link tutor). This can then be used at the final interview as a reminder as to what was required.

Action plan guidelines

- Identify the learning outcomes/competencies that have not been met.
- Write explicit behavioural objectives, i.e. what the student should know or do.
- Identify the learning activities required to reach these targets.
- Identify what support is required.
- Identify the timescale and review dates.
- Specify what evidence of achievement is required.
- Document and sign, and each take a copy.

- **Provide support and resources.** Having identified deficits and formed an action plan, the mentor is responsible for offering support and resources as identified in the action plan. The mentor will need to work closely with the student from this point onwards and continue to ensure that the student works with associate mentors to increase the objectivity of subsequent assessments.

- **Final interview.** If the student has been successful on placement, the final interview should be a cause for celebration. However, if the student has not succeeded, then it should once more be a tripartite meeting, to ensure its objectivity and fairness. This also serves to support both the student and the mentor. Should a student fail the placement, the meeting should create and record an action plan for future learning, so that any deficits can be subsequently identified and rectified.

Final interview . . . failure

It will be fairly clear ahead of the final interview that the outcome is not going to be a happy one, and this gives you time to ensure that it is managed in a professional manner. There are several things you need to take into account:

- Remember that in most cases the student will not be 'failing the placement', just not achieving all their competencies. In most cases, they can take these with an action plan into their next placement or have a special placement arranged for them to achieve those competencies.

- Ensure that you have discussed the student's placement with associate mentors.

- Ensure you have booked a quiet room and will have privacy.

- Ensure that it is a tripartite meeting with the link tutor.

Use the sandwich technique for breaking bad news. Ensure a positive opening and a positive and constructive ending.

- Be frank about the failed competencies and give clear guidance as to how they can be achieved. In a worst case scenario where the student has acted in a grossly unprofessional manner, this is especially important. The link tutor should help to reiterate this, thus underlining the importance of the failure.

- Allow the student to comment and give their views.

- Allow the student to express their sadness and concern. Support the student emotionally and validate and acknowledge their emotional state. Listen to them and support their determination to persevere.

(continued)

- Invite the link tutor to comment.

- Together, write a clear and achievable action plan for the student to take away.

- End with a reaffirmation of the student's positive qualities and your belief in their abilities. That you believe it is within them to redeem themselves should mean a great deal.

- **Student reaction and support.** To be told that you have failed the placement is unwelcome news to say the least. But done professionally and having adhered to the process outlined above, the news should not come as a shock to most students who will be aware that they have fallen short of the required standard. However, some will take the news personally, and feel aggrieved and angry or just shocked at the realisation that their future is in jeopardy. Students should be given time to take stock and mentors should allocate time and be prepared to allow the student to think about and discuss the bad news. The mentor needs to be prepared to deal with any emotions that may surface and allow the expression of those emotions, be they anger or sadness. The student needs to express their anger or sadness before they can enter into a rational discussion about the repercussions and any future action plan. It is never easy to deal with raw emotions but allowing and acknowledging them goes a long way towards helping the student deal with them and move forwards. If the mentor suspects that it will be an angry encounter, they may wish to organise some support for both themselves and the student by inviting the link tutor or other appropriate person from the university to the meeting. In the main, students are grateful for emotional support and any guidance as to how to move forwards.

Second-year student accepting appropriate criticism

At first I was a bit taken aback and about to get all defensive, but as he was explaining it to me I had to agree that he was right. He outlined quite clearly the goals we had set and the opportunities I had had to meet them. But he also said he believed I would reach them and that he felt I would make a great nurse. From that point on, we sat and talked about why I hadn't met them and worked out an action plan for me to work on. I have to admit I am a bit inflexible and stubborn and need to feel more comfortable with taking on advice and not dismiss it in a huff. If I'd been a bit more self-aware I'd have learnt.

A reflection upon supporting mentors and student

In my capacity as the practice learning team link tutor, I was asked by the mentor to meet with both themselves and the student in question. The mentor had expressed concern that the final-year student was unlikely to complete their placement outcomes by the end of the placement. The student had just completed their intermediate interview and had not really produced any significant evidence congruent with the level expected for semester 6. The staff were concerned that the student did not seem to appreciate the level they should be working at for this stage of their training. The meeting was difficult, as it was necessary to ensure that both the mentors and the student felt supported. The staff were faced with the possibility of failing the student and the student needed to feel that they were given the best possible opportunity to achieve their outcomes.

At the beginning of the meeting, the student was made aware that the mentor and staff team felt that with only 6 weeks to go there was little chance of the student being able to reach the required standard. A very frank discussion was facilitated where the student and staff were able to talk freely about the difficulties they had. Several elements were identified that required attention, including a much more detailed and thorough approach to gathering and presenting portfolio evidence of achievement.

A comprehensive action plan was agreed incorporating the student being much more proactive in relation to demonstrating competencies in clinical and communication skills. The need for a detailed action plan was vital to ensure that all concerned were very clear of what needed to happen to ensure the process was fair and robust. The student was also warned that there was a strong possibility that they might need a few extra weeks in order to achieve the outcomes, but was reassured that the clinical team were confident that the student could do it.

The student did need an extra 4 weeks and the staff kept in touch with me via email, but neither the student nor the mentors felt the need to arrange any further meetings.

Attitude

Poor attitude

A poor attitude is often a feature of poor student performance, and Duffy suggests that we should place more emphasis on attitude in assessing students. But what exactly is a poor attitude?

Evidence suggests that mentors are poor at failing students for reasons other than lack of knowledge or clinical competence. Often, despite evidence supporting an unprofessional approach and other 'attitudinal' problems, mentors will pass students because they have 'achieved all their outcomes'. There is a 'personal' element involved here, which makes it hard for us to question the attitude of another person. It is also less clear-cut and sometimes there is a vagueness about attitude that is hard to pin down and express precisely in words. Even where there is space to comment upon such in student placement documentation and which is not going to fail the student, mentors seem reluctant to comment. Duffy (2003) has identified this as a major failing.

Attitude

Often it is an unprofessional attitude, rather than any deficit in clinical skills or knowledge, that leads a student to fail a placement.

In relation to a student who appears unmotivated and uninterested and who does not seem to participate in the ward or team:

• What might be the reasons for this?

• What can a mentor do about it?

• Can you design any exercises related to your clinical area that would force the student to consider these aspects of their presentation, their professional role and responsibilities, and how others might perceive them?

There are competencies that can clearly be failed by students who display a 'poor attitude', show poor communication skills, are disrespectful, lack enthusiasm and motivation, and fail to work well within the team. Sometimes mentors fail to use these in relation to attitudinal problems.

Table 9.1 lists competencies which relate to attitudinal issues with suggestions for evidence students might be asked to produce to show achievement. It is by no means exhaustive. It represents a template for individual mentors to adapt to their own clinical area and locality. It also, by default, represents a list of good reasons to fail a student for not displaying these qualities.

Alongside the above there are quite clear essential skills at each progression point that students can fail if their attitude towards their clients and colleagues is poor. Mentors must begin to pay heed to these if the qualities of care and compassion are to remain key elements of the profession. To this end, these essential skills should be reviewed at the mid-point of each placement and clear guidance given to students who are not meeting the required standards.

Table 9.1 Competencies and evidence in relation to attitude

	Domain and competency	Student evidence
1.1	Practise with confidence according to The Code	Reflective writing regarding the NMC Code's clauses relating to respecting the client and cooperating with others in the team Discuss the principles of privacy, dignity, confidentiality and consent. Student conducts discussions relating to clients in a secure and private manner. Student demonstrates enthusiasm and motivation
1.2	All nurses must practise in a holistic, non-judgemental, caring and sensitive manner that avoids assumptions	Discuss your status as a visitor when in clients' homes Student seeks permission and gains consent Student uses appropriate communication skills in initiating dialogue Student acts in a respectful and professional manner
1.2	Recognises and respects individual choice	Discuss the rights of patients to refuse treatment Explore ways in which clients can be involved in their own care Discuss the Mental Capacity Act 2007 Student involves clients or carers in healthcare assessments, care plan reviews and decisions Demonstrates ability to adapt approach and communication skills to different clients
1.2	Challenge inequality, discrimination and exclusion	Recognises and respects the needs of the cognitively impaired Can discuss the nursing implications for a client living in poverty
1.3	Support and promote the health, well-being, rights and dignity of people, groups, communities and populations	Student respects the wishes of clients and actively seeks their opinions Student is non-judgemental in their approach Student can discuss a range of cultural and religious beliefs common in the local community Student is aware of a range of support services they can utilise to meet the cultural or religious needs of clients Student demonstrates a non-discriminatory approach to clients

(continued)

Table 9.1   (*Continued*)

	Domain and competency	Student evidence
4.4	All nurses must be self-aware and recognise how their own values, principles and assumptions may affect their practice	Student is able to demonstrate awareness of own learning needs Student sets goals for future learning Student responds positively to constructive criticism Student demonstrates good rapport with elderly clients, using appropriate language Student demonstrates good rapport with adolescent clients, using appropriate language Student is able to reflect upon the importance of communication skills in nursing care
4.7	All nurses must work effectively across professional boundaries, actively involving and respecting others' contributions	Student demonstrates a willingness to engage in the team Student is aware of support services and other agencies to whom clients may be referred Student can discuss the roles of other members of the multidisciplinary team Student undertakes insight visits to other team members' services Student is courteous and professional in dealings with fellow professionals

Source: NMC (2008b)

It is also possible to highlight in more detail aspects of the NMC Code of Conduct that relate to attitudinal issues, as shown below.

Treat people as individuals

- You must treat people as individuals and respect their dignity.

- You must not discriminate in any way against those in your care.

- You must treat people kindly and considerately.

Collaborate with those in your care

- You must listen to the people in your care and respond to their concerns and preferences.

- You must make arrangements to meet people's language and communication needs.

- You must share with people, in a way they can understand, the information they want or need to know about their health.

Ensure you gain consent

- You must ensure that you gain consent before you begin any treatment or care.

- You must respect and support people's rights to accept or decline treatment and care.

- You must uphold people's rights to be fully involved in decisions about their care.

Maintain clear professional boundaries

- You must refuse any gifts, favours or hospitality that might be interpreted as an attempt to gain preferential treatment.

- You must not ask for or accept loans from anyone in your care or anyone close to them.

- You must establish and actively maintain clear sexual boundaries at all times with people in your care, their families, and carers.

Work effectively as part of a team

- You must work cooperatively within teams and respect the skills, expertise, and contributions of your colleagues.

- You must consult and take advice from colleagues when appropriate.

- You must treat your colleagues fairly and without discrimination.

Act with integrity

- You must demonstrate a personal and professional commitment to equality and diversity.

Accountability and responsibility in practice

Mentors are accountable to a range of people in undertaking their mentoring responsibilities.

The students

Mentors are accountable to students in many ways, such as enabling their learning, assessing them fairly and providing honest, constructive feedback. Mentors also have a professional duty to students to maintain standards of supervision and assessment. Students need to know what they need to improve upon to allow them to develop and increase their knowledge and skills. Having done so, the student's success is ultimately the mentor's responsibility. Modern clinical assessment dictates that it is the role of the student to provide the evidence to persuade the mentor that they are competent, even though the final decision lies with the mentor. The principles of adult learning dictate that the student is responsible to a large degree for their own learning. The mentor must ensure that students are aware they are largely responsible for any failure on their part.

Experienced mentor's reflective discussion with novice mentor

By giving a true judgement, mentors will fulfil their responsibility to students, who will be sure of their actual learning needs for the future, and not be misled into false impressions, believing they are competent, when in actual fact they may be failing.

They may not see it at the time, but by failing an incompetent student you are protecting them from future harm. By passing an incompetent student, you place them at risk of making mistakes and at worst causing a tragedy. There is also the possibility of being struck off the register and the trauma of legal proceedings and even a custodial sentence if found guilty. Thus, failing an incompetent student has a protective function not just for the patients but for failing students themselves.

Ourselves

Accountability to the self is not immediately obvious, but mentors are accountable for their decisions in practice when mentoring a student.

Biting off more than they can chew!

Occasionally, a student will agree to perform a procedure or undertake a task which they are not yet competent at, without close supervision. By doing this, patient care is compromised and both student and mentor are placed in a difficult position.

What reasons are there a student might do this?

Unlike the mentor, the student is not professionally accountable because they are not on the professional register. However, both the student and mentor are legally accountable for their practice. The mentor is accountable for students' level of supervision and support. A student who says they can perform a task is in legal terms saying, 'I am competent' and thus they become legally accountable. The mentor is also legally accountable for a student's actions when they let them undertake a procedure. In the eyes of the law, the mentor will be deemed to have assessed that student's competence as satisfactory for the task in question. For this reason, the mentor must be as sure as possible of the student's level of competence prior to letting them perform any clinical procedure. This underlines the importance of getting to know your student early on in the placement in order to be able to judge their level of competence.

Worst-case scenario

A mentor agrees that a student can perform a procedure without really having a good idea of their level of competence. Things go wrong, the client is injured, and it all ends up in court. The student is held legally responsible for their actions, as they agreed to do the procedure. The mentor is also held legally responsible because they let the student do it. A good solicitor will be asking awkward questions, including: 'Upon what evidence did you make your assessment that the student was competent to undertake this procedure?'

Being aware of the student's level of competence becomes more important as the student progresses through training, because as they do so the mentor should be delegating more tasks and allowing the student to do more and more. At the same time, the mentor will be reducing their level of supervision, as the student moves towards unsupervised and competent practice. It's a 'Catch 22' situation: you need to give the student more experience and freedom, but ultimately you are still their supervisor and accountable. Students vary enormously in their levels of competence regardless of what stage or year they are at. First-year students will vary from the young person straight out of school who has no care work experience, to the novice who is more mature and has worked as a nursing assistant for many years. You would expect the latter to be more competent, but this might not necessarily be the case. Similarly, it is easy to assume that final placement students are all but competent; such an assumption would be wrong and the mentor must still make a careful assessment of competence in order to decide what level of supervision to give each individual student. As a mentor, then, you are accountable for the standards of care your students deliver.

The nursing profession

As mentors, we have a professional duty of care to fail incompetent students. The main reasons for failing students are when they do not provide sufficient or relevant evidence of achievement, or when they act in an unprofessional or unsafe way. However, as explored above, attitude and professionalism are areas of student assessment that are often neglected. The implications of continuing to ignore the error of leniency are potentially severe in relation to the mentor's responsibilities to the profession, the public, and our clients. There is also a partly selfish element that is worthy of inclusion here: as mentors we are safeguarding the standing of our own profession. We act as the profession's gatekeepers and we should be asking ourselves, 'Is this person worthy of joining and representing my profession?' By failing to fail, we are devaluing our own profession and its standards.

Experienced mentor's reflective discussion with novice mentor

Making valid assessments helps the mentor to meet their accountability to their own profession, as they can distinguish between those students who will make good nurses and those who will bring the profession into disrepute.

Our employer

We are accountable to our employer because it is usually a condition of our employment that we act as mentors to student nurses in training as well as to junior staff.

The professional body, the NMC

We are accountable to our professional body in many ways but directly in relation to student nurses, as the Code of Conduct states that we have a duty to pass on our knowledge and 'facilitate students and others to develop their competence'. Mentors are also accountable to the NMC for the judgements they make regarding those students.

The public

Mentors are responsible for ensuring that student nurses do 'no harm' to clients during their clinical experiences. Patients are put at risk when incompetent nurses are passed. Ultimately, such decisions could result in deaths. It is the quality of patient care that is at stake, and thus it is this that the mentor is ultimately accountable for.

NMC requirements

A final word about the importance of keeping records. The NMC (2006) suggests that it is important for mentors to keep records (an audit trail) to support their decisions: 'Mentors must keep sufficient records to support and justify their decisions on whether a student is, or is not, competent/proficient' (NMC 2006, p. 34). Obviously, this is more important in the case of a failing student: mentors need to be able to show that they provided regular feedback and kept a record of such. There is usually an appropriate space within the student's Ongoing Assessment Record where such notes can be recorded.

Novice mentor

I have come to understand the importance of collecting robust evidence supporting my evaluation of a student's performance.

Supporting the mentor – or, helping the mentor survive a placement!

Much of the information in the preceding chapter will also be of benefit to the mentor in ensuring their continued faith in human nature and a willingness to mentor students. It is a rewarding experience but one that at times can appear thankless and lonely. It need not be so. Nevertheless, the mentor needs to be proactive in accessing the help and support on offer. It is a good policy to build robust links with your 'link' tutor. This relationship is crucial, especially when things do not go smoothly. One important aspect of the mentor's support is their own diligence in assessing the student early on and having a good grasp of their level of competence. Identifying issues early saves much anxiety all around and the proverb 'Strike while the iron is hot' comes to mind. Raise the issues as they arise, don't sit on them. But let the pattern emerge rather than reacting to a 'first offence'! Meeting your student regularly helps enormously; if you do not, you cannot become aware of their concerns . . . or deficits. The mentor's greatest source of support is their colleagues and it is worth remembering that it is not the mentor's student but the team's student. The mentor should ensure that the student spends time with as many colleagues as possible. This widens the body of opinion as to the student's competence and is thus more objective and should give confidence to the mentor when a student has failed to meet their competencies. The 'link tutor' or relevant contact from the School of Nursing or university should can also be invited to take part in the mid-placement interview if the mentor has any concerns. This ensures that the mentor is not acting in isolation and is supported in the process.

Another part of the mentor's 'survival kit' is in ensuring that the placement has good learning opportunities that are a whole-team responsibility. However, the mentor should have successive groups of students

(continued)

try to identify other opportunities and facets of the placement that could help them and their fellow students learn and progress. This helps students take on board that they, too, are responsible for their own learning. It is also worth reiterating that it is the student's responsibility to convince you that they have achieved their competencies, and no longer your job to convince them they have done so.

Finally, it is important to ensure that all nurses who are qualified to be mentors undertake some mentoring. If some nurses avoid taking on the role, this leaves an unfair burden on the shoulders of those who take the responsibility. If this is the case, it should be raised at supervision. If any mentors reading this are asking 'what supervision?', they need to be asking their managers about getting some!

Summary

This chapter has:

- Examined the reasons why some mentors fail to fail

- Described good practice in providing feedback

- Described how to manage and support a failing student

- Focused on the difficult area of attitude

- Examined the accountability and responsibility issues in relation to failing students

In the final chapter, we examine some common problems in relation to the role of the mentor and consider how a mentor can remain competent and develop their mentoring skills.

Further reading

Dolan, G. (2003) Assessing student nurse clinical competency: will we ever get it right?, *Journal of Clinical Nursing*, 12: 132–41.

Hays, R. (2006) *Teaching and Learning in Clinical Settings*. Oxford: Radcliffe Publishing.

Lankshear, A. (1990) Failure to fail: the teacher's dilemma, *Nursing Standard*, 4(20): 35–7.

Nicklin, P. and Lankshear, A. (2002) Methods of assessment, in P. Nicklin and N. Kenworthy (eds.) *Teaching and Assessing in Nursing Practice*, 3rd edn. London: Baillière Tindall.

Royal College of Nursing (RCN) (2004) *Guidance for Mentors of Student Nurses and Midwives: An RCN toolkit*. London: RCN.

Rutkowski, K. (2007) Failure to fail: assessing nursing students' competence during practice placements, *Nursing Standard*, 22(13): 35–40. This article provides an overview of the issues surrounding mentors' reluctance to fail students in practice.

Welsh, I. (2003) Passing bad students fails us all, *Nursing Times*, 99(1): 17.

Useful web resource

www.practicebasedlearning.org/students/docs/assessment/page08.htm
This is a useful web-based resource covering many aspects of teaching and learning.

References

Duffy, K. (2003) *Failing Students: A qualitative study of the factors that influence the decisions regarding assessment of students' competence in practice*. Available at: http://science.ulster.ac.uk/nursing/mentorship/docs/nursing/oct11/failingstudents.pdf [accessed 2 March 2014].

Duffy, K. and Hardicre, J. (2007) Supporting failing students in practice 1: Assessment, *Nursing Times*, 103(47): 28–9.

NMC (2006) *Standards to Support Learning and Assessment in Practice: NMC standards for mentors, practice teachers and teachers*. London: Nursing and Midwifery Council.

Nursing and Midwifery Council (NMC) (2008a) *Standards to Support Learning and Assessment in Practice: NMC standards for mentors, practice teachers and teachers*, 2nd edn. London: NMC.

Nursing and Midwifery Council (NMC) (2008b) *The Code: Standards of conduct, performance and ethics for nurses and midwives*. London: NMC.

Skinner, B.F. (1971) *Beyond Freedom and Dignity*. New York: A Knopf.

Watson, H.E. and Harris, B. (1999) *Supporting Students in Practice Placements in Scotland*. Glasgow: Department of Nursing and Community Health, Glasgow Caledonian University.

10 Maintaining competence and developing as a mentor

> **Key points**
>
> - Mentors must remain updated and have their competence reviewed every three years
> - 'Sign-off' mentors are responsible for the final practice competence judgement
> - Mentors need to be well supported when supervising and assessing students
> - The future mentor role will be increasingly interprofessional in nature
> - Being a mentor is both a rewarding challenge and a privilege

NMC (2008) Domains and outcomes for a mentor related to this chapter

Establish effective working relationships

- Have effective professional and interprofessional working relationships to support learning for entry to the register

Assessment and accountability

- Foster professional growth, personal development, and accountability through support of students in practice
- Be accountable for confirming that students have met, or not met, the NMC competencies in practice. As a sign-off mentor, confirm that students have met, or not met, the NMC standards of competence in practice and are capable of safe and effective practice

Evaluation of learning

- Participate in self and peer evaluation to facilitate personal development, and contribute to the development of others

(continued)

Creating an environment for learning

- Identify aspects of the learning environment that could be enhanced, negotiating with others to make appropriate changes

Context of practice

- Contribute to the development of an environment in which effective practice is fostered, implemented, evaluated, and disseminated
- Initiate and respond to practice developments to ensure safe and effective care is achieved and an effective learning environment is maintained

Evidence-based practice

- Identify and apply research and evidence-based practice to their area of practice
- Contribute to strategies to increase or review the evidence base used to support practice

Leadership

- Be an advocate for students to support them accessing learning opportunities that meet their individual needs – involving a range of other professionals, patients, clients, and carers
- Prioritise work to accommodate support of students within their practice
- Provide feedback about the effectiveness of learning and assessment in practice

Maintaining competence

The NMC (2006) *Standards to Support Learning and Assessment in Practice* dictate that mentors must demonstrate their ongoing knowledge, skills, and competence as mentors and that this should be reviewed and assessed at triennial reviews. This is to be achieved by updating. The NMC requires placement providers to make provision for the annual updating of mentors so that mentors can:

- Maintain knowledge of current NMC-approved programmes
- Discuss the implications of any changes to the NMC requirements
- Have an opportunity to discuss issues related to mentoring, assessment of competence, and fitness for safe and effective practice

The obligation for mentors is to access this and other forms of updating so that they can demonstrate to the NMC and their employers how they have maintained their knowledge, skills, and competence. As part of their continuing professional development (CPD), qualified nurses should maintain and update their professional portfolios or profiles. Many will have compiled a portfolio as part of their mentorship course, and this could be added to with a section relating to updating.

SWOT analysis

It is advisable at this time that the mentor undertake another SWOT analysis. The importance of such analyses was discussed earlier and in order to maintain and improve our competence as mentors, these are useful tools to audit the level of that competence. All three variations mentioned previously will be useful, namely a SWOT analysis of the clinical area you support, a SWOT analysis of your own mentorship, and asking a student you have mentored to undertake a SWOT analysis of your mentorship of them. Use all three of these to develop an action plan and prioritise your areas for development.

Triennial review

This is a review and assessment of the mentor's ongoing competence as a mentor. Mentors will have to provide evidence that they are meeting the NMC mentor criteria and requirements. The triennial review is undertaken by the placement provider and is usually achieved via a form of appraisal or as part of ongoing supervision. In order to remain on the register, the NMC (2006) requires that mentors must have:

- Mentored at least two students in the last three years

- Undertaken annual mentor updating that included face-to-face meetings with other mentors to explore common issues

- Explored with others issues of validity and reliability when assessing practice in challenging conditions

- Mapped their mentorship development against the NMC standards

- Met the requirements to remain on the local mentor register

Mentor updates

In the past, there was a lack of specific guidance as to what should constitute an update. Updates were supposed to have been undertaken on a 'regular' basis but the content was largely left unspecified. Anecdotal evidence suggests that many mentors did not (and still do not) update regularly because of the pressures of work in particular, since patients must come first. Placement providers are now responsible for compiling and maintaining a register of mentors who will be reviewed every three years and that review will require them to have undertaken annual updates. The NMC (2009) now stipulates that annual updating must include:

- Review of NMC-approved programmes
- Overview of any recent changes
- Curriculum changes
- Support mechanisms
- Discussion of any NMC changes to requirements
- Discussion of mentoring and assessment of competence issues
- Problem-solving/trouble-shooting
- Sharing ideas for teaching sessions

Other useful content for mentor updates includes:

- Reviewing student documentation
- Reviewing portfolio evidence
- Recapping student interview needs/stages
- Reviewing levels of competency
- Essential skills clusters
- Triennial review
- Sign-off mentors
- Supporting students with a disability
- Reviewing supporting a non-achieving student

More recently, the NMC (2009) has provided guidance on the ways in which updating can be achieved, suggesting that it should be ongoing rather than an annual event. It also suggests other ways in which updating could be achieved, such as shadowing experienced mentors and undertaking literature reviews. Other useful methods are online updates and mentor update workbooks. *The Nurse Mentor and Reviewer Update Book* (Murray et al. 2010) provides useful advice on maintaining competence and providing evidence of such.

Evidence for portfolio

A wide range of evidence can be collected to demonstrate updating and maintenance of competence as a mentor. These should then be mapped to the NMC competencies for mentors. They include:

- Certificate of attendance at mentor updates
- Reflection on issues raised at mentor updates
- Action plan for implementing new ideas in mentoring
- Re-evaluation of clinical learning environment
- Identifying new learning opportunities
- Developing essential skills cluster teaching packages
- Involvement in educational audit
- Updating clinical area profile/student welcome pack
- Updating educational resources
- Showcasing evidence-based practice in the clinical area, e.g. via notice boards
- Evidence of student induction into area
- Reflecting upon difficult/successful mentoring scenarios with learning points identified (e.g. student demonstrating unsafe practice, student demonstrating unprofessional behaviour, the underachieving student)
- Anonymous action plans for non-achieving students
- Anonymous preliminary, intermediate, and final interviews
- Re-evaluation of validity and reliability of assessment methods
- Reading of relevant articles and learning points identified
- Evaluation of professional/statutory reports
- Shadowing an experienced mentor
- Contributing to/developing a mentors' newsletter
- Witness statements from students and associates
- Reviewing and acting upon student evaluations of placement and learning
- Teaching plans and feedback from teaching
- Undertaking a literature review
- Evidence of educational liaison with other multidisciplinary team members

- Links with School of Nursing, evidence of education/placement meetings attended

- Updated SWOT analyses

Evidence-based practice

It is crucially important in modern nursing that practice is underpinned with evidence. A good definition of evidence-based practice (EBP) is that of McKibbon (1998, p. 399): 'EBP is an approach to health care wherein health professionals use the best evidence possible, i.e. the most appropriate information available, to make clinical decisions for individual patients.' He argues that this builds upon the practitioner's clinical expertise and adds to the knowledge pool. It ensures that decisions are made based both on evidence and patient need and preference.

The following examples of evidence can be used to demonstrate that a mentor meets this mentor competence:

- Professional updating by training and workshop attendance

- Conference attendance

- Undertaking research in practice

- Evidence-based practice initiated/shared

At the heart of these and an essential aspect of implementing EBP is the ability to undertake a literature search.

Literature searching and appraisal – the stages

1. Identify a clinical question or problem that you want to find the answer to.

2. If you are unfamiliar with the process of electronic searching, arrange yourself a tutorial with the hospital or university librarian.

3. You will need to decide which databases are most relevant for your question. Good nursing databases include CINAHL (the Cumulative Index to Nursing and Allied Health Literature), Psychinfo, British Nursing Index, Medline, and ASSIA (Applied Social Sciences Index and Abstracts). Google Scholar is an increasingly useful staring point if you are unsure. These search engines give you access to peer-reviewed articles and papers, which means that they have been scrutinised and reviewed by experts in the field and are therefore robust.

(continued)

4. You will need to narrow down your search to stop you getting swamped and focus in on the most relevant material. The use of 'key' words and limiting the search will be of enormous help here and is a key skill. Useful limits to set may include: English language only, from a particular year onwards, published literature only.

5. You will next need to critically appraise the material you have gathered to ensure it is reliable and valid. Good questions to ask here include:

   - Is the person qualified to do the research, i.e. an expert in the field?

   - Was the sample size sufficiently large?

   - Is the sample representative, i.e. sufficiently similar to your clients?

   - Was the methodology appropriate?

   - How were the data collected?

   - How were the data analysed?

   - Who funded the research and is there any suggestion of bias due to self-interest?

   - When was it written, is it still current?

   - Does the discussion reflect the results?

   - Was it peer-reviewed?

6. Before implementing the change, you will need to ask yourself whether it will work for you in your specific setting. Other considerations include whether it is cost-effective, if there any drawbacks, whether you have the skills, and if it requires extra training. The most important thing, however, is whether the change fits in with your client's needs and preferences.

7. Finally, you will have to evaluate its effectiveness and the outcomes. This will entail devising an assessment tool to measure the improvement. This is important, as there is little point in going through all the above stages if you are unable to tell whether it has made any impact.

Publications

Aveyard, H. (2010) *Doing a Literature Review in Health and Social Care*, 2nd edn. Maidenhead: McGraw-Hill.

Ellis, P. (2013) *Evidence-based Nursing Practice*, 2nd edn. London: Sage/Learning Matters.

McKibbon, K.A. (1998) Evidence-based practice, *Bulletin of the Medical Library Association*, 86(3): 396–401.

(continued)

Web resources

www.nice.org.uk – National Institute for Health and Clinical Excellence
www.sign.ac.uk – Scottish Intercollegiate Guidelines Network – evidence-based guidelines for Scotland
www.library.nhs.uk – NHS health and social care resources and evidence
www.casp-uk.net – Critical Appraisal Skills Programme – tools for critiquing articles and research

Sign-off mentors

In 2006, the NMC introduced the concept of a 'sign-off' mentor so that the final judgement about a student nurse's capability to practise safely and effectively is made by a mentor who has experience and who has fulfilled additional mentorship criteria. All students entering training since September 2007 are required to have been finally assessed by sign-off mentors or practice teachers. Sign-off mentors have to meet certain additional NMC requirements to undertake the role (see below). The role of the sign-off mentor, then, is to judge whether the student has met the competencies for entry to the register and pass their decision to the School of Nursing and Midwifery or university. This is usually recorded on a separate page in the student's Ongoing Achievement Record (OAR).

- Pre-registration nursing students can only be signed off by the mentors assessing them in their final placement.

- Students on specialist practice programmes leading to a recordable qualification are required to be assessed by sign-off mentors (or in certain instances, practice teachers).

- Student midwives have to be supported throughout their training by mentors who have met the additional sign-off criteria.

- Student specialist community public health nurses must be supported and assessed by practice teachers who have met the additional sign-off criteria.

To be a sign-off mentor, a nurse or midwife must be identified as such on a local register and according to the NMC they must be:

- On the same part of the register as the student they are assessing

- Working in the same field of practice

- Clinically current and up to date

The NMC also states that the sign-off mentor must:

- Understand the programme requirements and assessment procedures for the students

(continued)

- Understand the NMC registration requirements

- Understand their accountability to the NMC for their decisions as to whether a student passes or fails

- Have been supervised in signing off a student at least three times by an existing sign-off mentor

The importance of the role of the sign-off mentor, then, is in confirming that the student is a safe and effective practitioner, who has completed their practice outcomes, and can be recommended to the NMC for registration. The sign-off mentor, via the student's OAR, has access to the student's placement records over the three years and can, if necessary, contact previous mentors. The responsibility for this final practice competence judgement used to lie with the educational institution, but now it lies with the sign-off mentor. To achieve sign-off mentor status, a prospective sign-off mentor must be supervised in signing off students on at least three occasions. The first two of these can be achieved by a variety of methods, including simulation, role-play or using interactive e-resources. These can be achieved as part of an approved mentor preparation programme. The third occasion must be with a student undertaking an NMC-approved programme under the supervision of a sign-off mentor (NMC 2010).

The NMC states that, 'Sign-off mentors must have time allocated to reflect, give feedback and keep records' (NMC 2006, p. 34) when mentoring final placement students. However, this 'protected time' is currently just one hour a week per student, which, one could argue, does not reflect the responsibility attached to the role.

Support for mentors

The NMC suggests that mentors have access to support and supervision to help them in their role and especially at times of having to make difficult decisions such as failing students. The NMC also recognises that support should foster the mentor's ongoing development. The obvious support mechanism is that of other, more experienced mentors. The other major form of support has traditionally been that of the 'link tutor', but the role varies widely across educational institutions. The role of the 'link tutor' in relation to supporting the mentor with a failing student is especially important and has already been examined. Many placement and education providers have developed specialist mentor support roles to provide mentors with updates and practical support. Other areas have grouped placements together to form teams; the mentors from these teams and the educational representatives meet regularly to discuss placement issues, update each other, and feed back student evaluations. The following is an example of one such team, which aims to combine mentorship issues with specialist clinical issues, acting as a support mechanism for mentors, students, and clinicians.

Practice learning teams: an experience

Birth

The university introduced practice learning teams (PLTs) to act as a replacement for the link tutor system of providing educational support to clinical placements for students undertaking pre-registration nursing courses. It was suggested that the link tutor system was not working effectively due to increased workloads of the tutors and the sheer number of students out on placement. Some clinical areas did not have dedicated link tutors and the methods tutors used to provide such links varied across the placement areas. Initially, the PLTs were set up geographically, with teams across all specialties meeting together regularly throughout the year to discuss common concerns regarding mentorship and student placements. However, the older adults mental health teams chose to set up their own, specialty-based PLT. This was for three main reasons:

- Much time at geographically based PLTs would be spent discussing student concerns not necessarily related to older adults' mental health placement experiences. The fear was that older adults' issues would be low on the other clinicians' agendas.

- There was also a realisation that meeting regularly as a specialty group would help to bring about cohesion among the older adults mental health teams, which was perceived as being lacking.

- It was also felt that the PLT could provide a forum to address wider practice issues related to the specialty but not primarily related to student educational needs. Indeed, it was felt that it would be foolish not to discuss major factors affecting the quality of service delivery to older adults while meeting together.

Membership of the PLTs is open to anyone with an interest. Each placement area identifies a PLT rep who is the core contact but meetings are open to all staff, including healthcare assistants and students. The team was split into two because of the size of the county and they meet twice a year with an additional annual conference.

Role

The roles of the PLT have become numerous over time, but the core features are as follows:

- Develop effective partnerships between the higher education institutes and the clinical placement areas

(continued)

- Provide support for students in practice
- Develop practice-based learning
- Foster practice development to improve the learning environment
- Support practice staff in their mentoring and assessment of students
- Provide mentor updates and advice
- Facilitate practice placement educational audit
- Review placement allocation
- Develop learning resources
- Forum for sharing good practice
- Problem-solving workshop
- Promoting practice-based research
- Facilitating student evaluation of placement and its feedback to the clinical areas
- Formulate action plans to address concerns
- Foster practitioner involvement in school-based teaching and university staff involvement in practice
- Mapping of learning opportunities available in clinical areas to the NMC
- Competencies students have to achieve
- Compiling student placement profiles

The annual conference is now a highly thought of and sold out away day, with any places not taken by staff quickly taken by students. The conference is an opportunity for staff to make a presentation at conference; students are encouraged to do so also. It is a great opportunity for the whole team across the county to meet together and network, and reaffirm the feel of a team. Each year the conference sets itself a task of building something tangible that will benefit students. In the first year, we achieved a mapping of all competencies to learning experiences in older adult mental health placements. The second year led to a list of 'creative learning experiences for students' with many excellent innovative ideas emerging from the practitioners, mentors, and students. The PLT is now in its sixth year.

Mentors should consider the benefits of joining forces with other similar specialist areas to form teams, such as that described above, to enhance support mechanisms and the student learning experience.

The other obvious form of support is clinical supervision, and mentors should access and use such support in relation to their mentoring activity as well as clinical activity. Mention should also be made here of healthcare support workers, whose value has been outlined elsewhere; here it will suffice to point out that by helping with students, they are also supporting the mentors in teaching and making assessment decisions.

NMC advice

A very useful source of advice and support is the NMC advice service, advice@nmc-uk.org. Here you can email the NMC or ring them (0207 333 6556) with any enquiries you have with regard to students, mentorship, and nurse education.

Common mentorship problems

In the previous chapter, we explored how to help failing students turn it around. It is also useful to explore at this stage some of the other practical mentorship problems and dilemmas mentors will come across. While suggestions are made for action and ideas, it remember that each student is an individual and each circumstance will be just that bit unique and as such each will need a slightly different approach to its solution. The first port of call should be that you seek guidance from an experienced mentor who will invariably have met with the situation before. Below are some common situations.

Too many students

The ward appears to regularly get allocated a large number of students and at times it seem like there are too many for the number of mentors you have and the limited number of learning opportunities available.

This can often happen, especially if it is an essential placement area. You should discuss the situation with your team to decide if there are ways of coping with this number. It may be that by using the full range of shifts and weekends you can spread the students out and make the situation manageable. Check the last educational audit and look up the recommended number of students it cites. If your allocation is regularly over this, then discuss the situation with the link tutor who should be able to reduce the numbers to a more manageable level. This is especially important if you have a limited number of mentors. Having too many students will necessarily dilute the placement experience, as the students

(continued)

will have to spread out the learning opportunities between them. The placement then becomes educationally unsound. As clinicians, we also need to be wary of having too many students, as it can become difficult to adequately monitor so many people safely. There will be times where too many students render the placement clinically unsafe and you have a duty as a nurse to identify this and rectify it. Clinical areas sometimes change quite rapidly and it may be that because of being exceptionally busy or through having unprecedented levels of staff sickness, leave or shortage, you have to request a reduction in student numbers. If a mishap occurred through being unable to safely supervise a student nurse, the legal responsibility for that mishap would lie with the mentor for not taking steps to rectify the situation.

Good friends

The two students you are currently mentoring want to work on the same shifts all the time.

There may not be enough mentors to allow two students on the same shift and learning opportunities need to be shared out, which is best achieved by students working opposite shifts. A regular feature of student feedback relates to placements being overcrowded with students and the suggestion that they have to 'fight' over learning experiences when they occur. Working apart also allows students to experience working with a wider range of other nurses and professionals rather than co-working with their friend. To allow for peer support, they could be rostered together for one or two shifts a week and for them to have some sort of group reflective supervision session. Should they protest, seek the involvement and advice of the link tutor.

The academic student

A bright student is always going to the library or is frequently on the computer and is primarily focused upon coursework.

This can be a common scenario as coursework assignments and passing them are high up most students' agendas. It may be that much is at stake and the student is worried about failing. You will need to sit the student down and have a frank discussion as to the purpose of the placement, emphasising that they are there to learn from the placement. Time management might be an issue and this can be talked through, helping the student to plan out their leisure time more effectively to incorporate time for study. You can still occasionally discuss the student's academic work with them in order to support them, but you should ensure that they are aware of their altered priorities while on placement. Students can access computers for legitimate placement-based work such as checking

(continued)

the evidence base for a procedure, and this should be encouraged as long as it doesn't take them away from the clinical experience too often. A student who spends much time on the computer might also be 'hiding' behind it. An open and honest chat to try and identify the reasons might unearth plausible ones such as high levels of anxiety on a first placement, or fear of failure. If you don't engage clinically, you can't get anything wrong! Identifying such reasons and giving appropriate support and guidance should help the student to more fully engage in the experience.

Unprofessional behaviour

This can come in many guises, including poor timekeeping and inappropriate dress. At its worst, it can be offensive behaviour and a disciplinary issue. Your current student has poor attendance and timekeeping, they never inform anyone or report sick, and seem to turn up whenever they like. What are mentors' responsibilities here? Is it a fitness-for-practice issue? What factors might be the cause? What will you do?

There is an obvious need to have a frank discussion with the student. Point out clearly what it is that you want them to stop doing and exactly what it is that you want them to start doing. Seek out any explanations such as childcare difficulties or stress and work out a mutual way forward that supports the student but also addresses their professional responsibility. It may be that you have to negotiate with them to have some time off in order to overcome the immediate crisis or problem. While discussing their professional responsibilities, identify for them the competencies these behaviours relate to. Reiterate the Code of Conduct and important issues such as reliability, and sickness and absence reporting procedures. Document discussions and write an action plan with goals clearly identified. Also clearly identify the competencies that they could fail to achieve. Repetition of the behaviour after it has been highlighted is a fitness-for-practice issue and the School of Nursing should then be involved, both to support the mentor and help the student understand the gravity of the behaviour.

A tripartite intermediate interview should formalise the issue and result in a clear action plan to work upon. Gross unprofessional behaviour, such as any form of abuse, should result in the mentor informing their immediate manager and the student being sent away from the ward until the matter is investigated and resolved. The School of Nursing should be informed immediately. Most schools will have their own fitness-for-practice guidelines and committees to deal with students acting unprofessionally either in the school or out on placement. A gross abuse is likely to result in the student being dismissed from the course and at worst the matter could be reported to the police. If a patient is involved, they may wish to make a formal complaint and this should be facilitated. Thankfully, however,

(continued)

most unprofessional behaviour is born of ignorance and usually a student will respond to the mentor pointing out the error of their ways, but the advice given must be concise and given in a manner that reiterates the seriousness of the event.

Unsafe practice

A student who used to be a nursing assistant performs an aseptic procedure with little regard for hygiene and compromises the sterile field. On pointing this out, they argue that that was the way the nurses did it on the ward they worked on before.

Again, a discussion is required here. Discuss the evidence base for doing the procedure the correct way and identify the aspects of bad practice the student has shown. Make this a focus of their placement experience over the next few days or weeks and work with them to show them the correct procedure. Unsafe and poor practice can occur for a variety of reasons other than simply not knowing better. Some students are over-confident and have an inflated idea regarding their own levels of competence and a mentor should be wary here. This could well be the case with the ex-nursing assistant who feels that they are already experienced. Be wary, too, of novice students trying to take on too much in order to impress and pass. The mentor needs to judge the student's level of competence early in the placement, for safety reasons, as we have explored in Chapter 9. There might be a need here to offer support to the student, who may be finding it difficult to get used to the change of role from nursing assistant to student.

As with the unprofessional behaviour scenario, there may be instances when the unsafe practice is so harmful that the student has to be asked to leave the placement until the matter is investigated. The School of Nursing should be informed and they will undertake their own investigation. The placement may also need to formally investigate the occurrence if patient care has been compromised. The student's mentor needs to handle this carefully and remain supportive of the student. The mentor should advise the student to write down their version of events as soon as possible.

Unmet outcomes

There are certain competencies a student cannot get on this placement.

This is quite common on some very specialist placements. The difficulty is usually overcome by arranging visits to other clinical areas for a shift or two where the competencies can be met. If your area has not mapped the competencies to learning experiences, this is something the team should consider doing as a matter of priority. Such a mapping document

(continued)

would identify what a student would have to do in that clinical area to meet those competencies. In this case, it might well identify any other areas the student should visit in order to achieve them.

Occasionally, through no fault of the student or mentor, there will be no opportunity for a student to achieve some outcomes. In this case, an action plan should be drawn up which the student can take to their next placement and share with their new mentor at induction.

Poor recording

The student's written reports are poor and contain many errors to the point that they could be misleading.

Have a confidential chat with the student to suggest the possibility of them being dyslexic. Let's assume that this is the case rather than laziness or carelessness, in which case the advice for the unprofessional behaviour and unsafe practice scenarios will be relevant. A student will likely find it hard to admit to being dyslexic, especially if they believe they will be asked to leave the course. The student might well be in fear of telling the School of Nursing. Discuss the possible risks around patient safety and the duty of professional responsibility and thus the need to be honest and seek help. Reassure the student and point them in the direction of the local support mechanisms. Use the strategies outlined in Chapter 8, 'Helping students survive a placement', to help them overcome the problem. Offer them ongoing support and reassurance that they can still succeed.

Lack of motivation

The student appears to be uninterested and unmotivated, they make no attempt to become part of the team.

This lack of apparent enthusiasm can arise for a variety of reasons and we must recognise that students are people first and students second. There may be personal reasons and problems at play and the student should be given the opportunity to discuss them. The student should be offered support if this is the case but reminded about their professional responsibilities. If the personal reasons cannot be worked around, then the School of Nursing should be involved. A lack of enthusiasm often occurs when other-field students find themselves on a short placement in an area of nursing they have no interest in. In the specialty of older adults' mental health, we are occasionally presented with a student who displays the behaviour as mentioned above. The student has no interest in mental health and informs us that they also 'don't do' older people. Nothing short of a rude awakening is called for here, but a humanistic and professional rude awakening of course. The student is displaying a lack of insight and in danger of missing a vital opportunity. In this case,

(continued)

we would point out to them that one in four people will suffer with serious mental health problems at some stage in their life. We would ask them to reflect upon the mental health needs of patients in adult nursing settings who are trying to cope with life-threatening injuries and diseases, coming to terms with loss of limbs and other handicaps, and trying to make sense of a diagnosis that clearly means that their life is shortened or at serious risk. Depression often goes undiagnosed in 'general' nursing settings; anxiety is an obvious accompaniment to being in hospital, however minor the complaint. The more the student nurse can learn about these issues and how to spot depression and anxiety, the better able they will be to do something about it. This may be a referral or just simply giving the patient the time to talk about their fears. Mental health placements can give adult nursing students an insight into these areas and also give them the skills to help and recognise the problems. Similarly, mental health students on adult placements have much to learn regarding good practice in clinical nursing skills and an appreciation of the mental health needs of the physically ill. Returning to the older adults mental health student, the great majority of clients of both the NHS and private care are likely to be over the age of 65. In addition, a great many of these people are likely to be confused for a wide range of reasons and a significant number will have a form of dementia. The need to pay attention to the placement and milk it for all it is worth soon becomes apparent to the unenthusiastic student once this is pointed out. While I have used older adults' mental health as an example, you will be able to come up with your own reasons why a student needs to pay attention to your specialty.

Some problems to ponder

A mentor will come across many other scenarios during their careers, to which there will need to be a clear response. While the advice on how to deal with a problem may be similar in many cases, there will always be some variation and the need to respond individually to each different student and scenario.

The poor student and the tired student

A student always arranges their shifts around the part-time job they have, as they are finding it hard to survive on the bursary. As a consequence, they are regularly turning up for work very tired and occasionally to the point of being barely fit for anything. How will you address this?

Consider also the student who over-enjoys their leisure time and is often late and tired but who, on the last two shifts, has had a strong smell of alcohol on their breath.

(continued)

The exclusive student

The student you are mentoring only wants to work with you and arranges that they are always on your shift. They are reluctant to work with health-care assistants and just seem to hang onto your shadow. How would you address this?

Poor professional boundaries

A young male student is clinically very good but is recklessly and openly flirting with the female patients not much older than him. What is the best way to handle this?

Recent developments

Interprofessional learning

Interprofessional learning is increasingly being embraced. Student nurses now undertake placements with a wide variety of other professions, reflecting the multidisciplinary nature of current practice. Mentorship courses are also beginning to be delivered across a range of professions such as nurses and operating department assistants. There is no reason why many other professions such as social work and occupational therapy should not access generic 'mentoring in health care' courses. Specific professional standards and requirements can be examined within such a course, which would also cover the generic aspects of mentoring and supporting learners in the workplace. Nurse mentors may well in future find themselves supporting a wider range of students from other disciplines who need to gain an appreciation of each other's role and place in modern health care. So nurses will need to understand the roles of others and also be able to support these others as they undertake work-based learning in their clinical environments. Wherever one works within nursing, a multiprofessional team is involved in supporting and enhancing the work nurses do. There is indeed an increasing blurring between the roles of those involved in the health and social care professions. Lack of professional collaboration has been shown to lead to a reduction in standards of care and poorer outcomes for clients in terms of quality of life and health. At worse, a lack of collaboration between nursing and other professions has led to high-profile tragedies such as the cases of Victoria Climbié, baby Peter, and Jonathan Zito, much of the blame for which can be put down to a lack of interprofessional collaboration and communication. There are many transferable skills between these professions and staff who are mentoring students from other professions should focus upon these. Mentors also need to know what stage the students are at and what the learning outcomes are for the placement. The bonus of accommodating such students is that they will often approach practice from a different perspective and this can be very enlightening.

Interprofessional working

Think about colleagues from other professions and services with whom you have to liaise, even though it may just be via telephone, and make a list. It will be longer than you thought.

Having compiled the list, arrange a visit or meeting to talk with these other colleagues in order to get a better understanding of what exactly it is that they do.

If possible, arrange for these other professionals to accept student nurses on insight visits if not already doing so.

Preceptorship

Preceptorship and mentorship are closely linked. The NMC suggests that qualified nurses who have at least a year's experience should support newly qualified nurses. The role is similar to that of an experienced mentor supervising a student mentor and will be one that many nurses are beginning to undertake at the same time as they are becoming mentors. Like mentors, preceptors should be willing and keen to share their knowledge. The two roles are linked, as having supported students during training the mentor could eventually find themselves supporting those same students during this major transition as they become familiar and get to grips with their qualified role. The roles of preceptors include facilitating new registrants, providing them with feedback on performance, support, action planning, teaching, and using the same skills and knowledge as within the mentor role. It seems logical, because of the similarities in role and continuity between the roles, that preceptorship be included as an element of mentorship courses.

e-learning

The pace of change is forever increasing, especially in the field of information technology, and education needs to continually embrace this. Mentors and nurses in general need to keep up to date with such changes and embrace them if they are not to be left behind. Younger generations of students are more likely to be familiar with a wider range of IT. Much current face-to-face teaching could well disappear with content being accessed electronically and remotely in many different formats. Electronic mentor updates and online mentor courses might become the norm with electronic portfolios and computerised student documentation the order of the day.

Regional variations

The Scottish approach to mentor preparation is along similar lines to that in England but is much more highly structured than in England and Wales. NHS Education for Scotland (2007) published the document *National Approach to Mentor Preparation for Nurses and Midwives: Core curriculum framework*. This was designed to ensure that all mentor preparation courses throughout Scotland met the NMC standards outlined in the 2006 *Standards to Support Learning and Assessment in Practice*.

NHS Education for Scotland sought to develop a national approach to mentor education that eliminated much of the variety of previous approaches adopted by higher education institutions. This new approach is delivered over 3 months as 10 days of 'learning effort', of which 5 days are protected time and 2 must include face-to-face contact. Budding mentors must demonstrate achievement of NMC mentor outcomes via a portfolio that has a prescribed format and is highly structured and comprehensive. There is a set core curriculum with 3 main areas of focus:

- Learning

- Professional accountability and relationships

- Assessment

There are set scenarios and focused activities to work through that are mapped to the NMC mentor outcomes, and for this reason it is well worth a read as it is a source of very good ideas for evidence of achievement of the NMC competencies.

Nursing and Midwifery in Scotland: Being fit for practice (NHS Education for Scotland 2008) is a report of the Evaluation of Fitness for Practice Pre-registration Nursing and Midwifery Curricula Project, a review of nurse education in Scotland and is a useful read in relation to what it has to say about practice education and mentors. It acknowledges the 'excellent' support given to students by mentors but highlights that there is a cost to mentors in balancing their responsibilities to both patients and students. One of the report's recommendations is that mentors be given support in relation to time and professional development to undertake their role effectively. The response of NHS Education for Scotland, who commissioned the report, was to reiterate the praise for mentors: 'mentors are the mainstay of pre-registration education and provide a high quality service' (Lauder 2008, p. 2). However, their response shies away from the 'time' element of support. The report suggests that the positive impact of mentorship is so strong that further means of recognising and rewarding mentors should be considered. 'We believe the best way is by . . . providing appropriate preparation and development opportunities, and by offering ongoing support' (Lauder 2008, p. 12). More encouragingly, it talks of incorporating mentorship into a structured clinical education career framework.

The situation in Wales is laid out in the 2002 document *Fitness for Practice: All Wales Initiative: Mentor preparation* published by the National Assembly for Wales. The mentor preparation programme here is 5 days over 6 months with set theoretical and clinical learning outcomes based upon the *Advisory Standards of Mentors and Mentorship* (UKCC 2000). The trainee mentor is then assessed evaluating a student's progress in practice against set criteria.

The mentor's role in fostering dignity and respect in care

Recent reports such as the Francis Report (2012), The Willis Commission on Nurse Education (RCN 2012), and the Keogh Review (2013), highlight among other things some deplorable staffing levels and subsequent failures in care especially with regard to patient dignity and respect. Although nurses cannot be blamed for the low staffing levels nurse mentors find themselves in, an increasingly important role is trying to uphold the values of good nursing care. In the face of the many pressures of modern nursing with diminished resources, it is the nurse mentor's role to pass on to students a working practice that encompasses both expertise and a respect for the patient and their dignity. Role modelling such behaviours is a vital aspect and powerful influence in eradicating these aspects of care failure.

The future!

The National Nursing Research Unit published a report in November 2012 entitled *Sustaining and Managing the Delivery of Student Nurse Mentorship: Roles, resources, standards and debates*. Commissioned by NHS London, its remit was to examine the 'Hinterland' of the delivery and receipt of nurse mentorship. The report gazed into a crystal ball and examined some of the key issues for the future. In terms of the current situation, it acknowledged the increased use of online learning as part of mentorship courses alongside the variability in nurses obtaining study leave to attend such courses. It remarked upon the importance of the high visibility of link lecturers in supporting mentors and confirmed that the relationship between link lecturers and practice staff was 'the "glue" that held the system together'. However, it acknowledged that the demands upon link lecturers' time were making this increasingly difficult to achieve. It concluded that mentors were doing a good job, 'often in challenging circumstances'. Sign-off mentors, for example, are partially meeting the one hour a week protected time by using their own time. The report concluded that widespread debate is required among all concerned and one key aspect is whether mentorship should be developed as a specialist pathway with dedicated time added to the role, thus providing a career pathway into nurse education. The recommendations of the Willis Commission (RCN 2012) into nurse education are a fitting place to end, as they include the recommendation: 'Employers must ensure mentors have dedicated time for mentorship . . . Mentors must be selected for their knowledge, skills and motivation; adequately prepared: well supported; and valued, with a recognized status.

Summary

There are many changes and many challenges facing the nurse mentor today. There is an ongoing battle for recognition of the undoubted value of the role and an urgent need for this to be addressed in terms of adequate protected time for mentorship. Despite the undoubted pressures and extra work being a mentor entails, it remains one of the most rewarding aspects of nursing and one of the most important. The rewards have been outlined in the Introduction and the importance is all too obvious in terms of ensuring safe and competent future practitioners. We should also regularly remind ourselves of the role of a mentor in safeguarding the reputation of our profession. The power to regulate who becomes a nurse and who does not lies in our hands and this is both a heavy responsibility and a privilege.

Further reading

Burns, I. and Patterson, I. (2005) Clinical practice and placement support: supporting learning in practice, *Nurse Education Today*, 5(1): 3–9.

Chapple, M. and Aston, E. (2004) Practice learning teams: a partnership approach to supporting students' clinical learning, *Nurse Education Today*, 4(2): 143–9.

Useful web resource

www.nes.scot.nhs.uk/practice_education/work/mentorpreparation/documents/
NatFrameworkMentoring-finalweb.pdf

References

Aveyard, H. (2010) *Doing a Literature Review in Health and Social Care*, 2nd edn. Maidenhead: McGraw-Hill.

Ellis, P. (2013) *Evidence-based Nursing Practice*, 2nd edn. London: Sage/Learning Matters.

Francis, R. (2012) *Independent Inquiry into Care Provided by Mid Staffordshire NHS Foundation Trust January 2005–March 2009*. Available at: http://www.midstaffsinquiry.com/assets/docs/Inquiry_Report-Vol1.pdf, http://www.midstaffsinquiry.com/assets/docs/Inquiry_Report-Vol2.pdf [accessed 2 March 2014].

Keogh, B. (2013) *Review into the Quality of Care and Treatment Provided by 14 Hospital Trusts in England: Overview report*. Available at: http://www.nhs.uk/NHSEngland/bruce-keogh-review/documents/outcomes/keogh-final-report.pdf [accessed 12 March 2014].

Lauder, W. (2008) *Nursing and Midwifery in Scotland: Being fit for practice*. The Report of the Evaluation of Fitness for Practice Pre-registration Nursing and Midwifery Curricula Project. Commissioned by NHS Education for Scotland. Available at: http://usir.salford.ac.uk/13929/1/Nursing_and_midwifery_in_Scotland_being_fit_for_practice_Final_report.pdf [accessed 2 March 2014].

McKibbon, K.A. (1998) Evidence-based practice, *Bulletin of the Medical Library Association*, 86(3): 396–401.

Murray, C., Rosen, L. and Staniland, K. (2010) *The Nurse Mentor and Reviewer Update Book*. Maidenhead: McGraw-Hill.

NHS Education for Scotland (2007) *National Approach to Mentor Preparation for Nurses and Midwives: Core curriculum framework*. Edinburgh: NES. Available at: http://www.nes.scot.nhs.uk/media/228890/mentor_prep_for_nurses_and_midwives_oct_2007.pdf.

NHS Education for Scotland (2008) *Nursing and Midwifery in Scotland: Being fit for practice*. NES Responses and Proposals following the Report of the Evaluation of Fitness for Practice Pre-registration Nursing and Midwifery Curricula Project. Edinburgh: NES.

Nursing and Midwifery Council (NMC) (2006) *Standards to Support Learning and Assessment in Practice: NMC standards for mentors, practice teachers and teachers*. London: NMC.

Nursing and Midwifery Council (NMC) (2008) *Standards to Support Learning and Assessment in Practice: NMC standards for mentors, practice teachers and teachers*, 2nd edn. London: NMC.

Nursing and Midwifery Council (NMC) (2009) *Additional Information to Support the Implementation of NMC Standards to Support Learning and Assessment in Practice*. London: NMC.

Nursing and Midwifery Council (NMC) (2010) *Sign-off Mentor Criteria*. Circular 05/2010. London: NMC.

Robinson, S., Cornish, J., Driscoll, C. Knutton, S., Corben, V. and Stevenson, T. (2012) *Sustaining and Managing the Delivery of Student Nurse Mentorship: Roles, resources, standards and debates*. London: National Nursing Research Unit, King's College London.

Royal College of Nursing (RCN) (2012) *Quality with Compassion: The future of nursing education*. Report of the Willis Commission. London: RCN.

UKCC (2000) *Standards for the Preparation of Teachers of Nursing and Midwifery*. London: UKCC.

Welsh National Assembly (2002) *Fitness for Practice: All Wales Initiative: Mentor preparation*. Cardiff: All Wales Policy for Pre-registration Nursing and Midwifery Education, Welsh Assembly Government.

Index